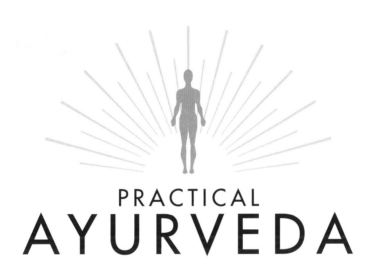

PRACTICAL
AYURVEDA

Sivananda Yoga
Vedanta Centre

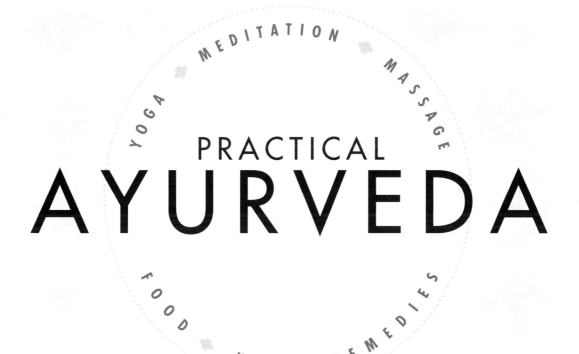

YOGA · MEDITATION · MASSAGE

PRACTICAL
AYURVEDA

FOOD · HOME REMEDIES

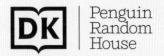

Editor Toby Mann
Senior Art Editors Emma Forge, Tom Forge, Saffron Stocker
Editors Anna Davidson, Tia Sarkar
Designers Amy Child, Vanessa Hamilton
Jacket Designer Saffron Stocker
Producer, Pre-production Tony Phipps
Producer Ché Creasey
Managing Editor Dawn Henderson
Managing Art Editor Marianne Markham
Art Director Maxine Pedliham
Publishing Director Mary-Clare Jerram

Illustrations Aurora Gritti, Keith Hagan
Photography Laura Edwards
Food Styling Maud Eden
Prop Styling Polly Webb-Wilson

First published in Great Britain in 2018 by
Dorling Kindersley Limited
DK, One Embassy Gardens, 8 Viaduct Gardens, London, SW11 7BW

The authorised representative in the EEA is
Dorling Kindersley Verlag GmbH. Arnulfstr. 124,
80636 Munich, Germany

IMPORTANT NOTICE

All participants in fitness activities must assume responsibility for their
own health and safety. If you have any medical conditions, consult with
your physician before undertaking any of the activities set out in this
book. The information in this book cannot replace sound judgement
when it comes to reducing the risk of injury, and you must take care.

Do not try to self-diagnose or self-treat serious or long-term problems
without first consulting a qualified medical practitioner as appropriate.
Do not exceed any of the recommended dosages. Always seek professional
medical advice if problems persist. If taking prescribed medicines, seek
medical advice before using home remedies.

CONTENTS

Foreword 6
Ayurveda and the four goals of life 8

YOU AND YOUR BODY 10
Ayurveda and the body 12
The three doshas 14
Reveal your constitution 16
The vata mind and body 20
The pitta mind and body 22
The kapha mind and body 24
How the body builds immunity 26

THE AYURVEDIC LIFESTYLE 28
A healthy lifestyle 30
A daily routine 32
Looking after your body 34
Self-massage 36
Step 1: Working towards a healthier lifestyle 40
Step 2: Achieving a healthier lifestyle 42
Step 3: Expanding your healthy lifestyle 44

MAINTAINING GOOD HEALTH 46
How to recognize problems 48
Pacifying vata 50
Pacifying pitta 52
Pacifying kapha 54
Strengthening agni 56

FOOD, DIET, AND RECIPES 58

The healing power of food 60
The six tastes 62
Sattvic diet 64
Consider vegetarianism 66
Herbs and spices 68
Ghee, sugar, and honey 70
The vata diet 72
Foods for vata 74
The pitta diet 76
Foods for pitta 78
The kapha diet 80
Foods for kapha 82
Supporting agni 84
Fasting for health 86
Cooking at home 88
Breakfast recipes 90
Lunch recipes 96
Dinner recipes 106
Dessert recipes 114

YOGA: ASANAS, PRANYAMA, AND RELAXATION 118

Ayurveda and yoga 120
Your yoga session 122
The yogic breath 124
Alternate nostril breathing 126
Lung purification 128
Neck exercises 130
Sun salutation 132
Single leg lift 136
Shoulderstand 138
Plough 140

Fish 142
Sitting forward bend 144
Inclined plane 146
Cobra 148
Child's pose 150
Camel 151
Tree 152
Crow 154
Spinal twist 156
Triangle 158
Active relaxation 160
Relaxation using autosuggestion 162

POSITIVE THINKING AND MEDITATION 164

Ayurveda and the mind 166
Monitoring the mind 168
The mind and the Self 170
Positive thinking 172
Refining our values 174
Meditation practice 176
The power of mantras 178
Karma yoga 182
The bigger picture 184

SEEING AN AYURVEDIC PRACTITIONER 186

Ayurvedic diagnosis 188
Your examination 190
Body treatments 192
Panchakarma 194
Ayurvedic medicines 196

HOME REMEDIES FOR COMMON AILMENTS 198

Treating common ailments by dosha 200
How to prepare home remedies 202
Remedies for common ailments 204
Remedies for respiratory tract ailments 206
Remedies for digestive tract ailments 208
Remedies for ailments of the eyes, hair, skin, and teeth 210
Remedies for trauma and musculoskeletal ailments 212

Glossary of terms 214
Index 215
International Sivananda Yoga Vedanta Centres and Ashrams 222
Acknowledgments 224

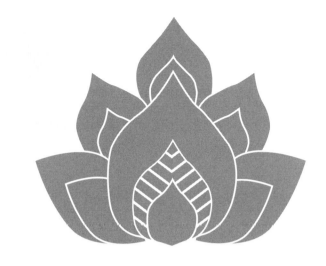

"A healthy person smiles and laughs, is cheerful and happy. Health is a gift from Mother Nature, the power behind life. Health is your birthright, not disease. It is as natural to be well as it is to be born."

SWAMI SIVANANDA

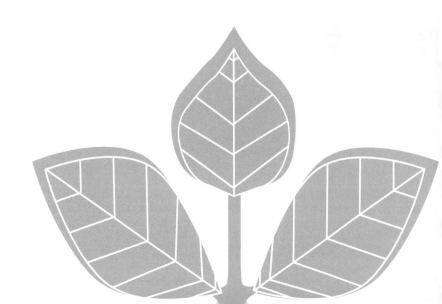

FOREWORD

Yoga and Ayurveda are sister sciences. Together, they show a way to live naturally and achieve radiant physical, mental, and spiritual health.

As one of the most important spiritual and healing traditions of the world, Ayurvedic and yogic scriptures describe the ethics and daily, monthly, and yearly practices of a healthy life; this covers topics including diet and exercise, as well as the use of the breath, senses, emotions, and mind. Their approach to meditation provides a step-by-step guide to complete peace and harmony – a balance of the mind and the heart – opening up the deeper potential of human awareness.

Practical Ayurveda follows the vision of Swami Sivananda (1887–1963), a renowned Indian yoga master and medical doctor who wrote over 200 books on all aspects of yoga as well as on Ayurveda.

It was Swami Vishnudevananda (1927–1993), an eminent disciple of Swami Sivananda, who, sent by his Master, brought the practice of yoga from India to the Western world. After establishing Sivananda Yoga Vedanta Centres in the Americas and Europe, Swami Vishnudevananda founded the Sivananda Yoga Dhanwantari Ashram, a unique training centre in Kerala, South India, where the practice of yoga and Ayurveda are combined.

The daily Ayurvedic routine allows you to gradually develop a healthier lifestyle. The food choices presented in this book work for both the individual person's constitution, and the practice of yoga and meditation.

While Ayurveda increases your prana (life energy) through diet, herbs, oils, and minerals, the practice of yoga and meditation teaches you to stabilize that prana in a more direct way – through postures, breathing exercises, deep relaxation, and meditation.

We hope that *Practical Ayurveda* will help you to heal yourself and to help you to manifest your full potential in body, mind, and spirit.

Swami Durgananda

Swami Sivadasananda

Swami Kailasananda

ACHARYAS OF THE INTERNATIONAL SIVANANDA YOGA VEDANTA CENTRES

AYURVEDA AND THE
FOUR GOALS OF LIFE

According to the classical Indian philosophy from which both Ayurveda and yoga originate, there are four goals of life. This book aims to help you focus on the goals of dharma and moksha.

What is Ayurveda?

Ayurveda means "science of life", and is comprised of a vast body of information about healthy living and treating disease. It covers areas of medicine that range from psychology to surgery, and paediatrics to geriatrics. Originally passed on through word of mouth, Ayurvedic knowledge was eventually written down in the ancient Indian language Sanskrit. Charaka, Sushruta, and Vagbhata are the authors of the three main classical Ayurvedic scriptures.

Ayurveda and yoga

In recent times, Ayurveda has expanded beyond India into the modern Western world, where its focus on health and overall wellbeing has been widely appreciated, and this has contributed to its growing popularity.

Ayurveda and yoga are two sister sciences that both come from the same philosophy. However, Ayurveda focuses primarily on the goal of dharma (living the right way), while yoga focuses primarily on the goal of moksha (enlightenment). Both are practical systems with a holistic perspective – people are seen as beings with a unified body, mind, and consciousness. Those who visit the Sivananda Vedanta Centres across the world will find both yoga and Ayurveda taught and practised there side by side.

DHARMA
(the right way of living)

Dharma is the principle of living one's life in a way that promotes inner and outer health and harmony, and in accordance with the universal principle of peace. Following dharma means to be truthful to one's nature, and acts from a sense of duty and respect towards it, rather than being driven by compulsive habits. This means living life with a sense of responsibility towards oneself, other people, and the world as a whole, and acting for the good of all. Ways to achieve this goal are covered throughout this book.

ARTHA
(material wealth)

A certain amount of money is needed to comfortably support oneself. Ayurveda and yoga place no judgement on the gaining of wealth, as long as it is done without causing harm to others, and that any abundance is shared.

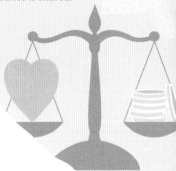

> *"Ayurveda is the knowledge of happy and unhappy, a good and bad life, and that which contributes to those four aspects."*
>
> CHARAKA

MOKSHA
(enlightenment)

Moksha means to overcome our limitations and become truly free within. This is a freedom from identification with the body and mind, and the realization that our true nature is a consciousness beyond those two things. This is a very difficult goal, and so the practices of hatha and raja yoga are devised to help one achieve it. Hatha yoga (pranayama, asanas, and relaxation) is covered in chapter five, while raja yoga (positive thinking and meditation) is covered in chapter six.

KAMA
(sensory pleasure)

Ayurveda and yoga recommend moderation when it comes to the pursuit of sensory pleasure. While it is beneficial to experience the positive influences of art and nature, over-indulging the senses can lead to addiction, frustration, and disease.

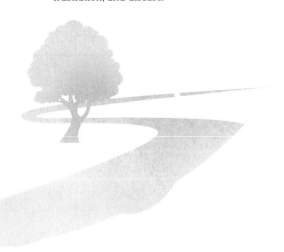

WHAT ARE
MY GOALS?

Sit in a comfortable position, close your eyes, and relax your body and mind. Detach yourself from the concerns of the past and future, and focus on the now. Ask yourself the following questions and let answers come from a deeper part of yourself:

- **What is my purpose** in life?
- **How can I contribute** to this world?
- **What are my values** and how can I uplift them?
- **What gives me** the greatest amount of contentment?
- **What is the next step** in my development?

YOU
AND YOUR BODY

"The three doshas, the seven dhatus, the three malas; these constitute the human body according to Ayurveda."

SWAMI SIVANANDA

AYURVEDA AND
THE BODY

There are four aspects of the body that need to be kept in balance in order to maintain good health – these are the doshas, the dhatus, malas, and agni.

Understanding the body

We must examine Ayurveda's understanding of how the body works in order to learn how we can maintain our health. This chapter will provide an outline of how the classical Ayurvedic scriptures describe the structures and functions of the body, and show you how your own body fits into that system.

A system of balance

Ayurveda teaches that the central principle of health is balance. Each of the four components here must be in a state of harmony – neither too strong nor too weak – for the body to remain healthy. This provides vitality by allowing greater capacity for prana (life energy required for all of the body's functions), and immunity from disease. The following pages will examine these components in more detail.

> *"The balance of the doshas is health, and imbalance is disease."*
>
> SWAMI SIVANANDA

Vata is the force of movement, activity, and sensation.

Pitta is the source of all transformative processes.

Kapha is the body's strength and stability.

DOSHAS *(energies)*

The three doshas are energies present within the body and mind. Maintaining the balance of each dosha allows the body systems to work effectively. For more information, see pp.14–15.

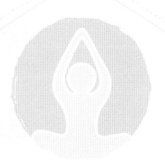

DHATUS *(tissues)*

The seven dhatus are the tissues that make up the body's physical form. Healthy dhatus allow the body to produce ojas, a form of energy that helps the body support prana (vital energy) and protects the tissues from damage. For more information, see pp.26–27.

AGNI *(fire)*

The main form of agni is the body's digestive fire. Healthy agni allows food to be digested so that strong tissues can be formed. It also prevents the build-up of ama, undigested food that acts as a toxin and leads to disease. For more information, see pp.26–27.

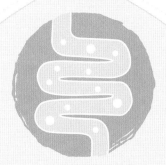

MALAS *(waste)*

The body's excretions – urine, stool, and sweat – are called malas. Passing them in a timely manner helps keep the body balanced, as otherwise they build up and can cause disease. For more information, see pp.26–27.

THE **THREE DOSHAS**

The doshas are energies that pervade the body and mind, each with different functions. All of the doshas can be found in everybody, but different people have more of some doshas than others – this determines a person's constitution.

Doshas, elements, and gunas

Vata, pitta, and kapha are the three doshas – three energies that are crucial to the healthy functioning of different body systems and the mind. Each dosha is made up of two of the five elements (air, earth, ether, fire, and water), the building blocks of all matter. The elements all have different characteristics ("gunas" in Sanskrit), and each has a principle – for example, water has the principle of fluidity. The doshas take on the characteristics of the elements from which they are made up. These characteristics define a dosha's nature and its role within the body.

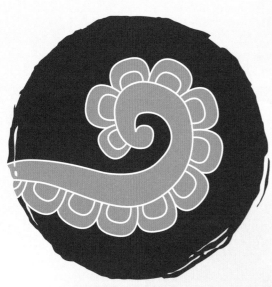

Vata *is the dosha of movement.*

VATA

Vata is made up of the elements air and ether. Air gives it characteristics such as mobility and dryness, while ether makes it subtle and light.

Vata is the most important dosha in the body and mind as it is the force of all movement (such as blood circulation) and sensation. The main seat of vata is the colon.

Vata's functions include:

- **Providing movement,** such as for breathing, circulation, nerve impulses, and the elimination of waste.
- **Providing all sensation** in the body.
- **Igniting agni.**
- **Supporting memory,** drive, and understanding.

Air element
(movement)

Ether element
(space)

PITTA

Pitta is made up of the elements fire and water. It takes on characteristics such as heat and sharpness from fire, and fluidity and oiliness from water.

In the body, pitta is the source of transformation (such as digestion) and provides internal heat. The main seat of pitta is the stomach and small intestine.

Pitta's functions include:
- **Digesting food** and fuelling agni.
- **Producing blood** and colouring the skin.
- **Providing intelligence** and self-confidence.
- **Providing sight.**

Fire element
(transformation)

Water element
(fluidity)

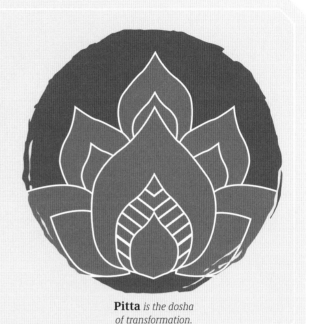

Pitta *is the dosha of transformation.*

KAPHA

Kapha is the dosha of earth and water. Qualities received by kapha from earth include heaviness and stability, and from water include oiliness and smoothness.

Kapha gives the body substance, strength, cohesion, lubrication, cooling, and immunity. It is also responsible for healing. The main seat of kapha is in the stomach and chest.

Kapha's functions include:
- **Providing moisture** to food in the stomach.
- **Providing strength** and cooling to the heart and the sensory organs.
- **Stabilizing and lubricating** the joints.
- **Providing taste.**

Earth element
(mass)

Water element
(fluidity)

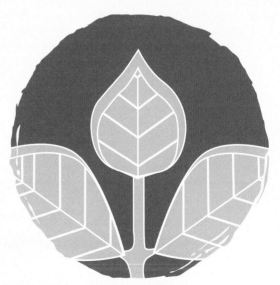

Kapha *is the dosha of substance.*

REVEAL **YOUR CONSTITUTION**

A person's constitution is determined by how much of each dosha they received at conception. This affects their body and mind. Knowing your constitution is key to health, as it is essential for understanding which lifestyle is best suited to you.

Self-assessment questionnaire

The following questionnaire will give you an idea of your constitution. However, it is not intended to replace the expertise of an Ayurvedic practitioner, who can give you a more accurate assessment.

For each question, choose the answer that best applies and give it one point. If more than one answer fits, give each half a point. If, for a particular question, you feel that the most appropriate answer has varied during your life, pick the answer that best fits the times when your life was stable or you were in good health.

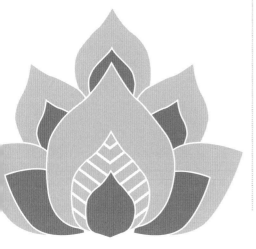

Q How would you describe your body?

a I have a slender, narrow frame with delicate bones, lean muscles, and well-defined veins and tendons.
b I have a medium frame with defined musculature.
c I have a sturdy, broad frame with large, solid bones. I can easily build up muscle and have a good layer of fat/padding beneath my skin.

Q How would you describe your joints?

a My joints are small. Occasionally they make cracking noises.
b I have flexible joints that are average in size.
c I have broad and firm joints.

Q How would you describe your skin?

a My skin is dry and thin, and can feel rough and cool to touch.
b My skin is soft and warm, and often moist.
c My skin is soft, moist to oily, cool and firm.

Q How would you describe your complexion?

a My skin can have irregular pigmentation. It tans easily.
b My skin has a healthy blush, and I have freckles or moles.
c I have an even complexion.

Q How would you describe your hair?

a My hair is fine and tends to be dry.
b My hair is fine and tends to be slightly oily. There may be signs of early greying or balding.
c My hair is lush, thick, dense, and slightly oily.

Q How would you describe your nails and lips?

a My nails are dry and brittle, and they can break easily. My lips are dry and quite thin.
b My nails are flexible and soft. My lips are pink and soft with a symmetrical shape.
c My nails are thick, smooth, and hard. My lips are pale, soft, and full.

Q Do you perspire much, and how strong is your body odour?

a I sweat very little.
b I sweat easily and in large amounts. My body odour can become strong and unpleasant.
c I do sweat, but I never notice much body odour.

Q Take a few deep breaths and then feel your pulse at your wrist. (For this it is best to be sitting down without having had any caffeine beforehand, or much stress or excitement.)

a My pulse is quick and soft. It isn't easy to define a definite rhythm – it moves like a snake.
b My pulse is strong and regular. It is neither fast nor slow, and feels like a jumping frog.
c I have a full, regular, and slow pulse that moves like a swan.

Q Do you enjoy doing exercise, and how often do you feel the need to move?

a I enjoy being active and find it hard to sit still. My movements are quick and I tend to fidget.
b I enjoy a good workout with a set goal and that requires precise and directed movements.
c I'm not always motivated to exercise, and find it easy and enjoyable to sit still for a good amount of time. I prefer to move slowly rather than quickly.

Q How much do you weigh, and how easily do you lose or gain weight?

a I tend to have lower weight than average and can lose weight easily.
b My weight is average. I can both gain and lose weight.
c I have a well-built body. I can easily gain weight, which is then hard to lose.

Q What sort of climate do you cope with best?

a I prefer it when the weather is hot, and I am very sensitive to the cold and the wind.
b I find it difficult to tolerate heat and direct strong sunshine. I prefer cooler temperatures.
c I can tolerate both hot and cold weather. Warm temperatures are best. Dampness and cold can become uncomfortable.

Q How would you describe your speech?

a I'm talkative and likely to speak fast. I'm liable to mumble, and maybe even stutter.
b I can be eloquent, and speak clearly and full of confidence. I have a strong voice.
c My speech is deliberate, measured, and steady. I have been told I sound soothing.

Q How is your sleep, and what time do you wake up in the morning?

a I'm a light sleeper. I tend to sleep less than average and to wake early in the morning.
b I sleep well and need about 6–8 hours of sleep.
c I sleep deeply and restfully. I like to sleep for a long time, and then find it difficult to wake up.

Q What types of food do you most like to eat?

a I prefer warm food and soups. I enjoy salty, sour, or sweet food.
b I prefer cold, sweet, and bitter food. Sometimes I enjoy salads and raw food.
c I prefer warm food. Pungent, dry, and light food suits me best.

Q How would you describe your hunger?

a My hunger varies, it can be either strong or weak. If I'm distracted, I can easily forget I'm hungry and skip meals.
b My hunger is strong, regular, and frequent. When I'm hungry, I need to eat right away.
c My hunger is regular, but generally weak. I'm often not very hungry, especially in the morning, and can make do with two meals a day.

QUESTIONS **CONTINUE**

Q **How would you describe your digestion, and how do you feel after eating a meal?**

a My digestion varies. I can feel full quickly, even though I was very hungry to start with.
b I have a strong digestion. My hunger often comes back relatively quickly after a full meal.
c My digestion takes time, it's better when I eat slowly. I can go a long time between meals without feeling hungry.

Q **How frequent are your bowel movements and what consistency are your stools?**

a My bowel movements often are less than once per day. My stools are dry and hard, and I'm liable to have constipation and wind.
b My bowel movements often are more than once per day. My stools are soft and copious, and they have a tendency to be loose or liquid.
c My bowel movements are regular, and my stools are well formed and in moderate quantity.

Q **How do you experience your emotions?**

a My mood can change quickly. I have strong likes and dislikes.
b When provoked, my emotions are strong. I can forgive easily.
c My mood is stable. I can sometimes come across as boring. Once I'm upset, I find it hard to forgive.

Q **How do you react to being stressed?**

a I get nervous and anxious, and I often feel insecure.
b I'm quick to anger and get irritated or impatient easily.
c I usually remain calm and level-headed. It takes a lot to get a reaction out of me.

Q **How do you find learning new things?**

a I learn very quickly if I focus.
b I have a sharp intellect and a good ability to focus.
c It takes time to learn new things.

Q **How would you describe your memory?**

a I have a very good short-term memory. My long-term memory is poor.
b I generally remember things well.
c Once I have learned something, I have excellent memory, especially in the long-term.

Q **How would you describe your thoughts?**

a I can think quickly on my feet and often have many ideas. My attention often wanders and I find it hard to focus on one single thing.
b My thoughts are clear and distinct, I prefer analytical thinking and planning.
c My thoughts tend to be thorough and methodical. I'm slow to develop new ideas. I like to stay on one topic.

Q **How well do you adapt to change?**

a I can adapt well to change – it suits my nature.
b I approach change as a challenge that I can master.
c I dislike change and find it hard to adapt. I prefer a steady routine.

Q **How are your energy and endurance levels?**

a My energy comes easily and in quick, short bursts.
b I have good energy and tend to push myself.
c I'm slow to get going, but have good endurance.

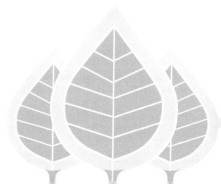

Your results

Count the number of marks you gave to a, b, and c respectively; **a stands for vata, b for pitta, and c for kapha**. The results will give you an idea of which doshas are dominant in your constitution, with the highest-scoring dosha being the most dominant.

Types of constitution

Most people have a constitution (NB not a "dosha") with two dominant doshas – these are indicated by the two highest scores. Some people have roughly equal amounts of each dosha in their constitution, so will have a fairly even score for all doshas. A constitution where one dosha is completely dominant over the two others (which are both equally low) is very rare.

Dosha characteristics

On the following spreads, you will learn about the full spectrum of possible characteristics imbued by each dosha. As we are all made up of a combination of the doshas, there may be some qualities on the page for your dosha that are not entirely true for you (even if you have a particularly high score for one dosha).

VATA (A)

If vata was your highest-scoring dosha or one of your highest-scoring doshas, move onto 'The vata mind and body' (pp.20–21). Here you can find out which qualities someone with a vata constitution is likely to have. Look for blue vata boxes throughout the book to find information specifically for those with vata as one of their dominant doshas.

PITTA (B)

If pitta was your highest-scoring dosha or one of your highest-scoring doshas, move onto 'The pitta mind and body' (pp.22–23). Here you can find out which qualities someone with a pitta constitution is likely to have. Look for red pitta boxes throughout the book to find information specifically for those with pitta as one of their dominant doshas.

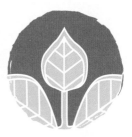

KAPHA (C)

If kapha was your highest-scoring dosha or one of your highest-scoring doshas, move onto 'The kapha mind and body' (pp.24–25). Here you can find out which qualities someone with a kapha constitution is likely to have. Look for green kapha boxes throughout the book for information specifically for those with kapha as one of their dominant doshas.

THE **VATA MIND** AND **BODY**

The vata constitution is predominantly characterized by movement. The vata mind is sensitive and creative. This leads to a slender build and active body functions, such as quick speech.

THE **QUALITIES** OF **VATA**

These are the characteristics of vata as described in the classical Ayurvedic scriptures. They help us understand the effect vata has on us.

moving
light
dry, cool
irregular
rough, fine
quick, formless

The vata mind

The influence of air and ether gives the vata mind properties of movement, lightness, speed, and irregularity (such as being able to understand and learn, but also being quick to forget). The diagram below provides more qualities associated with the vata mind.

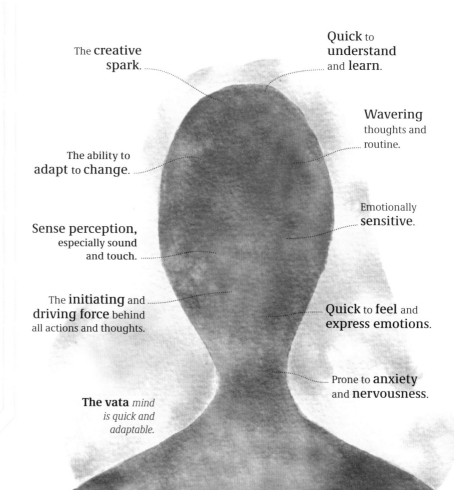

The **creative** spark.

Quick to **understand** and **learn**.

Wavering thoughts and routine.

The ability to **adapt** to **change**.

Emotionally **sensitive**.

Sense perception, especially sound and touch.

The **initiating** and **driving force** behind all actions and thoughts.

Quick to **feel** and **express emotions**.

Prone to **anxiety** and **nervousness**.

The vata mind is quick and adaptable.

The vata body

The influence of vata leads to a lean build and delicate structures. The vata body's functions tend to be active, unstable, and irregular. As functions fluctuate more readily than structures, they can be used as indicators to work out if vata has been increased or upset by your current lifestyle.

Light, short, and **easily disturbed sleep**.

Quick, **undirected movements** of **eyes** and **limbs**.

Can be **talkative** with **fast** and **soft speech**.

Hunger is sometimes **strong,** but can also be **absent**.

Thin, fine, **dry hair**.

Tendency to be **thin,** and to find it **easier** to lose than to gain weight.

Thin, dry, cool skin with early wrinkling.

Tendons and **veins** stand out.

Hard, **brittle,** thin **nails**.

Lean musculature.

Instable, delicate joints that can make cracking noises.

Long and **narrow limbs,** fingers or toes.

Prefers warm temperatures and finds the **cold** and **wind** uncomfortable.

Quick, **light,** and **changing movements**.

Susceptible to catching a **light cold**.

This is *the female vata form. Body structures are given on the left, and body functions on the right.*

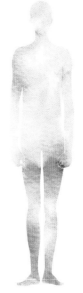

This is *the male vata form.*

THE **PITTA MIND** AND **BODY**

Clarity and heat characterize the pitta mind and body. This leads to an ambitious mind with a sharp intellect, and an athletic build with intense body functions, such as an active metabolism.

THE **QUALITIES** OF **PITTA**

These are the characteristics of pitta as described in the classical Ayurvedic scriptures. They help us understand the effect pitta has on us.

hot

sour, light

liquid, sharp

slightly oily

quickly penetrating

slightly foul smelling

The pitta mind

The influence of fire and water gives the pitta mind properties of penetration and transformation (such as a sharp intelligence and a proneness to anger). The diagram below provides more qualities associated with the pitta mind.

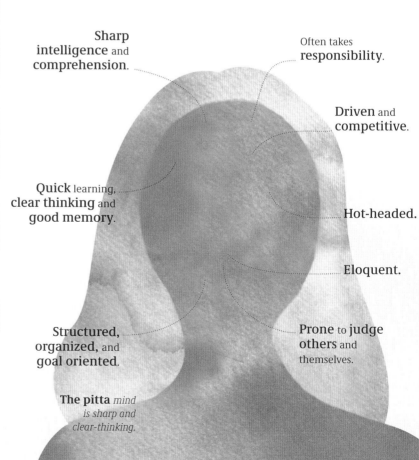

Sharp intelligence and **comprehension**.

Often takes **responsibility**.

Driven and **competitive**.

Quick learning, **clear thinking** and **good memory**.

Hot-headed.

Eloquent.

Structured, organized, and **goal oriented**.

Prone to **judge others** and themselves.

The pitta mind is sharp and clear-thinking.

The pitta body

The influence of pitta leads to a medium-sized build with flexible joints. The pitta body's functions are intense and sharp in nature. As functions fluctuate more readily than structures, they can be used as indicators to work out if pitta has been increased or upset by your current lifestyle.

The **head** becomes **hot** easily.

Clear, determined, and confident **speech**.

Symmetrical **features**.

Fine, **slightly oily hair**.

Sweats easily and profusely with a strong odour.

Average **weight**, finds both **losing** and **gaining** weight easy.

A very **active metabolism**, intense **hunger** and **thirst**.

Moist, oily, and **elastic skin,** occasional **freckles** and **moles**.

Elastic, shiny **nails**.

Well-**defined muscles**.

Intolerant to **heat**, enjoys the **cold**.

Flexible, elastic **joints** and ligaments.

Average-sized **limbs**.

Directed, **precise movements**.

Prone to **inflammation**.

This is the female pitta form. Body structures are given on the left, and body functions on the right.

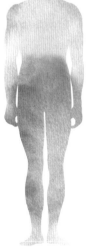

This is the male pitta form.

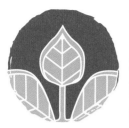

THE **KAPHA MIND** AND **BODY**

Structure and stability characterize the kapha mind and body. The kapha mind is patient and deliberate, while the kapha body has a sturdy build and slow-working body functions, such as a slow metabolism.

THE **QUALITIES** OF **KAPHA**

These are the characteristics of kapha as described in the classical Ayurvedic scriptures. They help us understand the effect kapha has on us.

cold
oily
heavy
stable, soft
slow, unmoving
sweet, viscous, sticky

The kapha mind

The influence of earth and water gives the kapha mind properties of stability and endurance (such as cool-headedness and good memory). The diagram below provides more qualities associated with the kapha mind.

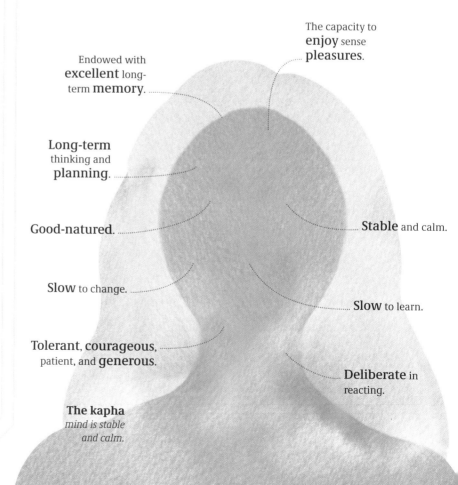

The capacity to **enjoy** sense **pleasures**.

Endowed with **excellent** long-term **memory**.

Long-term thinking and **planning**.

Good-natured.

Stable and calm.

Slow to change.

Slow to learn.

Tolerant, **courageous**, patient, and **generous**.

Deliberate in reacting.

The kapha mind is stable and calm.

The kapha body

The influence of kapha leads to a compact, sturdy physique with potential for muscle and fat build-up. The kapha body's functions are slow (sometimes lethargic) and stable. As functions fluctuate more readily than structures, they can be used as indicators to work out if kapha has been increased or upset by your current lifestyle.

Long, deep, **restful sleep**.

Slow, **soothing speech**.

Moderate amount of **sweat** that doesn't smell much.

A **slow metabolism**, doesn't have much hunger or thirst.

Thick, dense, **oily hair**.

Round, broad features.

Tends to **gain weight**.

Moist, **oily, cold, firm,** and thick skin.

Thick, strong **nails**.

Large, well developed **muscles**.

Firm, broad, and well-lubricated joints, firm ligaments.

Has **good endurance**.

Slow, **strong movements**.

Strong, sturdy, large **bones**.

Has **good immunity**.

This is *the female kapha form. Body structures are given on the left, and body functions on the right.*

This is *the male kapha form.*

HOW THE BODY
BUILDS IMMUNITY

Agni (digestive fire), dhatus (tissues), ojas (tissue protection), and malas (waste) are all vital for the body's health. All four are closely linked, and their health and function depend on each other.

Aspects of immunity

In Ayurveda, agni means "fire", and refers to the body's digestive fire. It is responsible for all processes of transformation, most important of which is building healthy dhatus.

The seven dhatus are plasma; blood; muscle and skin; fat; bone; nerve tissue and bone marrow; and reproductive tissue. They are created in a chain, with each digested by agni to produce the next. Food is digested to produce the first dhatu, plasma, then plasma is digested to produce blood, etc.

Ojas is created last in the dhatu chain, and so is often called the "eighth dhatu". It is a substance that supports prana (life energy) in the body and provides immunity from disease.

Malas refers to the body's excretions, such as urine, stool, and sweat. They must be eliminated efficiently to maintain the health of the body. The flow charts on the right show the effects of weak and healthy agni, and how this affects dhatus, ojas, and immunity.

Ama and weak agni

If agni is weak, the doshas are unbalanced, or malas are eliminated inefficiently, ama (undigested food) builds up in the body. It acts as a toxin and disrupts the body's healthy function. To prevent ama, maintain healthy agni through diet and exercise (see pp.56–57).

HEALTHY AGNI

The body is able to digest food, properly absorb its nutrients, and produce healthy dhatus. This means it can produce more ojas, providing more immunity and more capacity for prana.

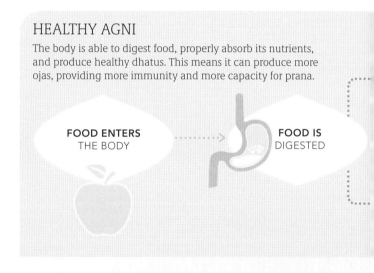

FOOD ENTERS THE BODY

FOOD IS DIGESTED

WEAK AGNI

The body cannot digest food properly. Undigested food is called ama (see left), and this builds up and causes disease. Unhealthy dhatus are formed and less or no ojas is produced.

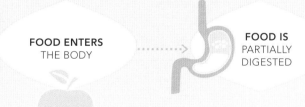

FOOD ENTERS THE BODY

FOOD IS PARTIALLY DIGESTED

"All disease occurs due to the disfunction of agni."

CHARAKA

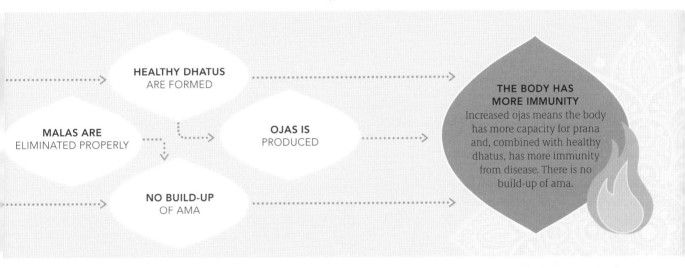

HEALTHY DHATUS
ARE FORMED

MALAS ARE
ELIMINATED PROPERLY

OJAS IS
PRODUCED

NO BUILD-UP
OF AMA

THE BODY HAS MORE IMMUNITY
Increased ojas means the body has more capacity for prana and, combined with healthy dhatus, has more immunity from disease. There is no build-up of ama.

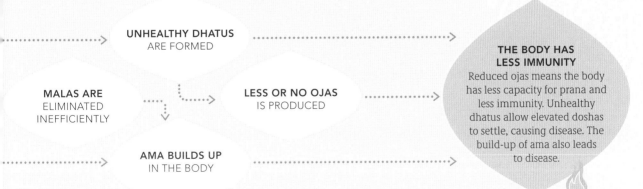

UNHEALTHY DHATUS
ARE FORMED

MALAS ARE
ELIMINATED
INEFFICIENTLY

LESS OR NO OJAS
IS PRODUCED

AMA BUILDS UP
IN THE BODY

THE BODY HAS LESS IMMUNITY
Reduced ojas means the body has less capacity for prana and less immunity. Unhealthy dhatus allow elevated doshas to settle, causing disease. The build-up of ama also leads to disease.

THE
AYURVEDIC
LIFESTYLE

"Health is the state in which you sleep well, digest your food well, are at ease and free from any kind of disease."

SWAMI SIVANANDA

A HEALTHY LIFESTYLE

The Ayurvedic lifestyle is based on three things: routine, moderation, and tuning in to the natural rhythms of the doshas and agni.

What is healthy?

Health is a positive state of happiness achieved through the normal condition of the doshas, dhatus (tissues), agni (digestive fire), and malas (waste), as well as a serene state of body, mind, and senses.

Ill-health starts with a dosha imbalance. First one or more of the doshas become "irritated" (a minor imbalance). If they are not pacified, they will increase until they are "elevated" (a more significant imbalance) and start to cause disease in the body. The build-up of ama (toxins), inefficient elimination of malas, and weak agni also contribute to poor health.

The information and lifestyle practices shown in this chapter should be performed by people of all constitutions at all times. Look out for boxes that provide information for those with a dominant dosha(s). Instructions on how to tailor your lifestyle to your personal needs will appear in the next chapter.

> *"Have faith in yourself; do the right thing; help others. This is the key to success, health, and happiness."*
>
> SWAMI SIVANANDA

ROUTINE

Performing healthy practices at the same time each day embeds them in your lifestyle. Your body will know when to prepare itself to wake up, digest food, and go to sleep. For more information about how adapting your daily routine can benefit your health, see pp.32–33.

MODERATION

Moderation provides balance to our lives and prevents over-indulgence. Most commonly, the road to ill health begins with a lapse in judgement. Even though we know better, we frequently choose to make unhealthy choices, most often in pursuit of sense pleasures. This might be overloading the stomach with an excessive meal and disrupting our sleep cycle by staying up too late and sleeping during the day, or suppressing natural urges to cry, yawn, or even go to the toilet.

NATURAL FLUCTUATIONS

The influence of the doshas on our bodies and the strength of our agni constantly change due to the time of day (see pp.32–33), our age, and the seasons (see below). We must tune in to these changes to keep to a healthy lifestyle.

PHASES OF **LIFE**

Make sure you take into account the strength of the doshas at each stage of life, as this will affect how much you need to balance them.

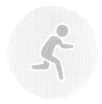

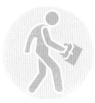

Childhood is the time of kapha. Children need kapha to grow, so it should be supported and not irritated.

Adulthood is the period of pitta. Your lifestyle should follow your dosha levels (see pp.48–49) and the influence of the seasons.

Old age is influenced heavily by vata, so make sure to be aware when it is accumulating so that you can pacify it.

THE **SEASONS**

The strength of agni and the doshas varies throughout the seasons. In the classical Ayurvedic scriptures, the seasons are described as winter, summer, and rainy, according to India's subtropical climate. These terms can be equated to the seasons of the world's temperate regions. Vata is also sensitive between the seasons, and may need pacifying.

In winter, vata increases and should be pacified. Eat a nourishing diet to satisfy growing agni. Kapha will accumulate, so try to keep warm.

In spring, the kapha accumulated in winter melts, producing allergy and fatigue. Make sure to reduce and eliminate this excess kapha.

The summer heat weakens agni and depletes energy. Pitta accumulates and should be pacified, especially if there is rain.

In autumn, vata again accumulates, which further weakens agni. Make sure that you strengthen agni during this period.

A **DAILY ROUTINE**

The strength of each dosha varies throughout the day, affecting how well our bodies perform different functions. To maintain balance, build your daily routine around when each dosha is strongest.

The daily rhythm of the doshas

The body and mind follow an internal clock – a cycle of 24 hours. At different times of the day, the doshas change strength, and with them their influence on the body and mind. By adapting your daily routine to these phases, you are keeping the doshas well balanced, ensuring they work effectively. For example, agni (digestive fire) is most active when pitta is strong during the daytime (10am to 2pm), so this is when you should eat your largest meal.

The daily rhythm of the individual doshas' strength influences our experience of the doshas within our bodies. For example, a person who has kapha as one of their dominant doshas may find it particularly difficult to get up during the time kapha is strong. This is because any natural heaviness from his or her constitution is added to by the extra strength of kapha at that time of day. It is therefore especially important for them to get up before 6am (during vata time), when the strength of vata counteracts their naturally high kapha levels, making them feel lighter.

Keeping to a routine

Regularity in your routine is essential. Getting up, eating, and going to bed at the same time each day will provide an ideal framework for a healthy life and a day full of energy. All of the body's processes will benefit from this regularity. For example, eating your meals at the same times each day means your agni will know to become active at those times.

Aim to go to bed at the latest at 10pm. The heaviness and inertia of kapha help induce restful sleep.

10pm

Agni is less active at this time, so eat earlier in the day to ensure you get restful sleep.

KAPHA

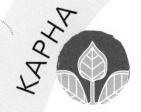

Avoid bright screens and use this period for calming activities, such as meditation or yogic breathing.

6pm

Dinner should be light, and is best eaten around 6pm.

VATA

Eating dinner before 6pm allows ample time for digestion before you go to bed.

2pm

This 24-hour clock *shows the periods of the day that each dosha is active, and what to do during each period.*

PITTA

The fiery energy of pitta can make it difficult to go to sleep after 10pm.

4–6am is called brahma muhurta. At this time harmonious vibrations boost the effects of yoga and meditation.

2 am

VATA

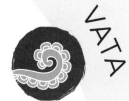

Get up before 6am to make the most of the energy and lightness provided by the strength of vata. This is a good time for meditation and yoga.

Agni is less active, as it is slowed down by strong kapha. Breakfast should therefore be light, or may even be skipped by those with dominant kapha.

6 am

This is the time when agni is most active, fuelled by the strength of pitta. Make sure to have your largest meal of the day at this time so that it can be properly digested.

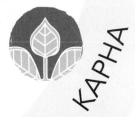

KAPHA

10 am

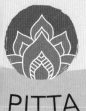

PITTA

SLEEP FOR **VATA**

Those of a vata nature need the most sleep, (about 8–9 hours each night). To help soothe restlessness before bed, they should have a hot bath or oil massage during vata time, then go to bed during kapha time to ensure restful sleep.

SLEEP FOR **PITTA**

People of a pitta nature need 7–8 hours of sleep each night. They benefit from turning off their screens an hour before going to bed. Calming breathing exercises and meditation after 6pm will help them get to sleep.

SLEEP FOR **KAPHA**

Those of a kapha nature only need about 7 hours of sleep. They should rise during vata time (before 6am) to get the best start to the day. If their kapha is balanced, they should have little problem getting restful sleep.

LOOKING AFTER **YOUR BODY**

Cleanliness is a key part of an Ayurveda, and there are many practices that are recommended as part of a healthy Ayurvedic lifestyle. Having a clean body will make you feel better and also be beneficial to your health.

A morning routine

Ideally, you should perform each of these practices every day, but practices that are new to you are best built into your routine gradually. To get an idea of where you can start, use the guide on pp.40–43.

"Health is wealth. Tune yourself with nature. Observe the laws of hygiene. Enjoy immortal bliss."

SWAMI SIVANANDA

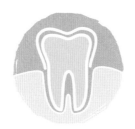

1 BRUSH YOUR TEETH

Use a toothbrush to thoroughly clean your teeth. You may want to use an Ayurvedic toothpaste. These contain herbs with antiseptic and anti-inflammatory properties, such as neem or cloves.

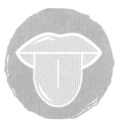

2 CLEAN YOUR TONGUE

Scrape away the coating on your tongue that accumulates nightly. Use a silver, copper, or steel tongue cleaner (not plastic), or your middle and index fingers. Start at the back and gently move to the front, repeating three to four times.

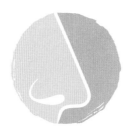

6 PERFORM NASYA

Apply plain sesame oil to your nostrils by dabbing a drop of oil onto your finger and massaging the inside of each nostril. This practice (called "nasya") keeps the nasal passage clear and alleviates headaches.

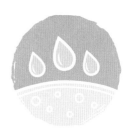

7 PERFORM OIL PULLING

Place 1–2 teaspoons of plain sesame oil or warm water in your mouth, and gently move the liquid back and forth for up to 5 minutes. Then spit it out. This practice strengthens your gums and reduces bacteria in your mouth.

"Have a glass of hot water early in the morning – it will help ignite agni, lubricate the body, and support bowel movements"

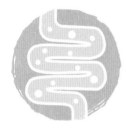

3 CLEAR YOUR BOWELS

It is best to have a daily bowel movement first thing in the morning. Timely and regular elimination of the waste products gives lightness to the body and prevents disease caused by ama (see pp.26–27).

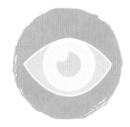

4 REFRESH YOUR EYES

Refresh and clean your eyes by dabbing your eyes and washing your face with cold water. This will remove any mucous or dirt that has built up in your eyes during the night whle you were asleep.

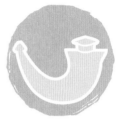

5 CLEAR YOUR NASAL PASSAGE

Use a neti pot to clear excess mucous from your nose and sinuses. Mix ½ teaspoon salt with 240ml (8fl oz) warm water, and pour it into one nostril using the pot. When done, blow out the remaining water from each nostril.

8 INHALE AROMAS

Light some incense (organic incense is best). Gently inhale the smoke to pacify kapha and ease morning heaviness. Scents that are recommended include sandalwood, rose, frankincense, and champa.

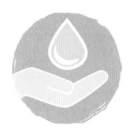

9 PERFORM AN OIL MASSAGE

Oil massages (see pp.36–37) are recommended for everyone. The simplest oil to use is sesame oil (good for vata and kapha). Those with pitta can use cooling coconut oil. For more about how to choose oils, see pp.38–39.

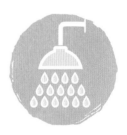

10 SHOWER OR TAKE A BATH

Ayurveda places great importance on cleanliness. Washing the body should be part of everyone's morning routine. In order to protect your hair and eyes, avoid using very hot water on your head.

SELF-**MASSAGE**

Massages are part of an Ayurvedic lifestyle due to their many benefits. Use these instructions to perform a self-massage at home, and at a time that suits you.

PHYSICAL **BENEFITS**

- **Nourishes** the body's dhatus.
- **Removes fatigue** from the body.
- **Promotes restful** sleep.
- **Relieves tension** in the muscles.
- **Boosts blood** circulation.
- **Protects against** ageing.
- **Pacifies** the doshas.

Performing a self-massage

A massage is best performed in the morning or late afternoon, but if needed, doing a massage any time is better than not doing one at all. Your stomach should be neither too full nor too empty. Sit on a warm, stable surface in a room that is around 25ºC (77ºF). Use more oil between the steps as required. If you are short of time, you can do only steps 1 and 2 as a simple alternative.

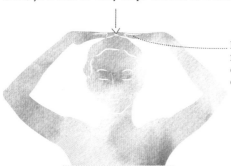

Press down firmly, without causing any discomfort.

1 **Take a handful of oil** in each hand and massage the top of your head using your open palms, then fingertips.

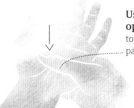

Use your opposite thumb to massage the palm of your hand.

2 **Massage each palm,** then interlock your fingers, gently tightening them and pulling your hands apart. Then do the same to your feet, massaging your soles and interlocking your fingers and toes.

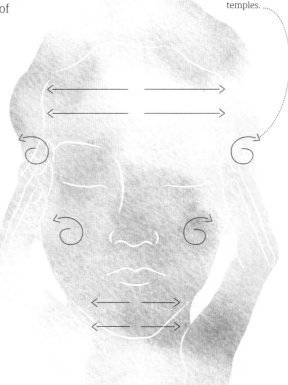

Use a circular motion to massage your temples.

3 **Massage your forehead** with horizontal strokes, your temples and cheeks with circular motions, and your chin with horizontal strokes.

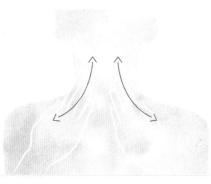

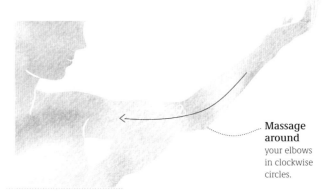

Massage around your elbows in clockwise circles.

4 **Now massage your throat,** neck, and shoulders with upward and downward strokes.

5 **Start on your shoulders** and stroke down your arms on the outside, stroking back up on the inside. Pay attention to the shoulder and elbow. While vata and pitta are soothed by strokes along the lines of the body hair, kapha benefits from emphasizing the strokes going against the lines of the hair.

"Pay your oil man and save your doctor fees."

TAMIL PROVERB

Massage around your knees in clockwise circles.

6 **Massage your legs** in the same way as the arms with both hands. Pay attention to the hips and knees. Strokes along the lines of the body hair soothe vata and pitta, while kapha benefits from emphasis on strokes against the body hair.

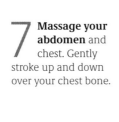

7 **Massage your abdomen** and chest. Gently stroke up and down over your chest bone.

Use a clockwise motion for your abdomen and chest.

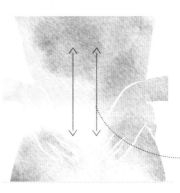

8 **Massage your back** and buttocks. Finish the massage with a long stroke from your heart to each hand, and from each hip to each foot.

Use firm upward and downward strokes on you back and butocks.

NOW MOVE ON TO
CHOOSING MASSAGE OILS

Choosing massage oils

Massages can be tailored directly to the needs of your body by choosing the correct massage oil. A system of balance dictates the effect of oils on different conditions. For example, pitta is hot and sharp, so the oils chosen to pacify elevated pitta are cooling and soothing (see the boxes right and opposite).

Dry powder massages

Oil massages are the most common form of massage. However, digesting oil rubbed into the skin requires strong agni, and so when agni is weak (such as when there is ama, fever, or infection), dry or dry powder massages are more appropriate. Dry massages simply use silk gloves rather than oil, whereas dry powder massages use a herbal paste. Dry powder massages are heating, stimulating, and dehydrating, making them beneficial for weak agni and excess kapha.

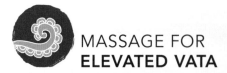

MASSAGE FOR ELEVATED VATA

Oil massage is one of the best and most effective treatments for vata. An oil massage with special vata oils or plain sesame oil is heating, reduces dryness and provides nourishment and grounding. A full body massage followed by a steam treatment is best, but if time is an issue, regular partial oil massages also work very well. If you have a tendency to vata imbalance, regular oil massage should be part of your routine.

To pacify vata, use these oils:

- **plain sesame oil** (heating)
- **almond oil** (warming and soothing)
- **olive oil** (heating).

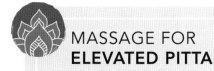

MASSAGE FOR ELEVATED PITTA

Oil massages with cooling or soothing oils like coconut or almond oil and special pitta oils pacify pitta. They provide grounding and calm, which counteracts pitta's lightness and sharpness. Pitta's highly active intellect gets a well-deserved rest with this full body sensory experience.

To pacify pitta, use these oils:

- **coconut oil** (cooling).
- **almond oil** (warming and soothing).

IMPORTANT NOTE

Oil massages should not be performed if you have ama (undigested food, see pp.26–27), fever, acute infection, or anaemia.

Dry powder massages should not be performed if you have skin irritation or rashes.

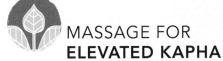

MASSAGE FOR
ELEVATED KAPHA

Stimulating massages which use dry powder, silk gloves, or heating oils such as special kapha oils or sesame or mustard oil give lightness and heat, which pacify kapha. They are especially effective if followed by a steam bath or dry heat.

To pacify kapha, use dry powder or one of these oils:

- **mustard seed oil** (very heating, do not use for the whole body, but just specific parts at a time)
- **plain sesame oil** (heating).

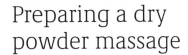

Preparing a dry powder massage

Mix together the following ingredients to prepare the powder for a massage.

- **300g (10oz)** chickpea flour
- **2 tbsp** dried basil
- **2 tbsp** dried sage
- **1 tbsp** neem powder (optional)
- **1 tbsp** shallaki powder (optional)
- **1 tbsp** Amalaki or Triphala powder (optional)
- **2 tbsp** finely ground rock salt

MASSAGE WHEN
AGNI IS WEAK

As it is difficult for the skin to digest oil when agni is weak, one must make careful considerations when performing a massage in these circumstances. Massages using dry powder, silk gloves, or specific oils can help stimulate agni in the skin.

Oils that stimulate agni in the skin are:

- **mustard seed oil** (very heating, do not use for the whole body, but just specific parts at a time)
- **Special, medicated, ayurvedic sesame oils** (heating).

"Oil massage slows ageing, removes fatigue and body aches, provides sound sleep and body strength, and prolongs life."

SWAMI SIVANANDA

AFTER A MASSAGE

Wipe off as much of the oil as you can with tissue paper immediately. Then remove the rest with soap or have a shower. Avoid exposure to the cold and wind, and take time to rest.

WORKING TOWARDS A **HEALTHIER LIFESTYLE**

If healthy living is new to you, then start here, using this three-step guide to work towards a full Ayurvedic lifestyle. Remember, regularity and moderation are key, and that it is best to introduce changes slowly so that they last.

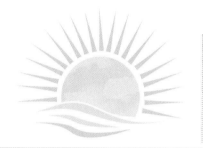
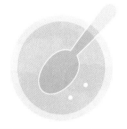
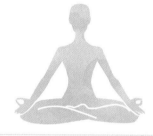

The start of your day

Try to get up 30 minutes earlier than usual. Then add one or two of the hygiene practices below to your morning routine.

- **Massage the top** of your head and then your feet with oil (see pp.36–39), and then shower.
- **Clear your** nasal passage and then clean your tongue (see pp.34–35).
- **Have a glass** of hot water before breakfast.

Food and mealtimes

Mealtimes are one of the most important aspects of an Ayurvedic lifestyle. Choose one of the suggestions below.

BREAKFAST
- **Try eating** a simple breakfast (especially if you aren't in the habit of having breakfast). Find inspiration on pp.90–95.

LUNCH
- **Have a warm** meal and take your time while eating.

DINNER
- **Replace salads** and raw foods with a warm, cooked meal.

Yoga and meditation

Performing a complete yoga and meditation session every day can feel like a big commitment. Start by doing the following.

- **Do a complete** yoga session once a week (see pp.120–63).
- **Do 5 minutes** of meditation every day (see pp.176–77).

Pick one of these things to introduce into your daily life.

- **Do 5 minutes** of abdominal breathing and body awareness each day (see pp.124–25).
- **Do 5 minutes** of positive thinking each day (see pp.172–73). Use the affirmation, "My heart is filled with compassion towards all beings".

WORKING TOWARDS HEALTH

Don't try to change every aspect of your lifestyle at once. Use this advice to build up healthy practices:

- **Start with one** or two aspects, perhaps those you are most motivated to change.
- **Don't try to change** anything that clashes with your duties at home or at work.
- **Make a plan** and note your progress. If you miss a goal, just go back to the previous step.

ADVICE FOR VATA

Those of a vata nature should try to:

- **Drink fewer** caffeinated drinks – try switching to green tea, which has a lot less caffeine.
- **Avoid eating** salads and raw food in the evening – try a warm soup instead.

Physical exercise

If regular exercise is new to you, use the following steps to build it into your daily and weekly routines.

- **Start slowly**, with 10 minutes a day, and add 1 minute each day.
- **Exercising in** the morning is best, but more important is being able to exercise at the same time each day.
- **If you miss** a day, just pick it up the next day – don't allow frustration to build.
- **See pp.50–55** to find out which form of exercise is best-suited to your constitution.

The end of your day

Sleep is often neglected in a modern lifestyle. Try to do the following things each night to get a more restful night's sleep.

- **Go to bed** 30 minutes earlier than usual.
- **Avoid using** your computer, television, or phone for at least 15 minutes before going to bed. Use this time for a period of quiet contemplation.
- **See p.33** to find out the best way for someone of your constitution to get a good night's sleep.

ADVICE FOR PITTA

Those of a pitta nature should try to:

- **Have a** late-afternoon snack of fresh sweet fruit every day.
- **Take 15 minutes** each day to cool down using active relaxation (see pp.160–61).

ADVICE FOR KAPHA

Those of a kapha nature should try to:

- **Do a** little extra exercise, such as walking up the stairs instead of using the lift.
- **Eat less** at night and start the day with an agni drink (see p.85).

STEP 2
ACHIEVING A HEALTHIER LIFESTYLE

You have already started to change your lifestyle and experienced the benefits, here is how you can improve on your progress and stay motivated. Aim to continue to add new practices and habits at the same pace.

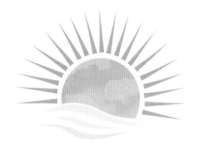

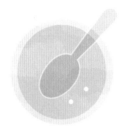

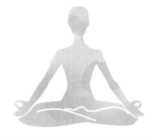

The start of your day

Aim to get up around 6am by setting your alarm 10 minutes earlier each fortnight. Gradually add the practices below to your morning routine.

- **Practise positive** thinking – wake up with a feeling of gratefulness towards all life (see pp.172–73).
- **Practise nasya** and oil pulling (see pp.34–35).
- **Perform a** self-massage once a week before you take a shower (see pp.36–39).
- **Drink one** or two glasses of hot water to have a bowel movement. (See pp.208–209 for home remedies that support bowel function.)

Food and mealtimes

Buy the basic spices (see pp.68–69) and eat one meal a day at the same time. You may want to work towards vegetarianism to increase sattva (see pp.64–67).

BREAKFAST
- **Adapt your breakfast** to your dominant dosha(s) (pp.90–95).

LUNCH
- **Prepare a simple** lunch, such as stir-fried veg (p.104), each morning, and bring it to work in an insulated lunch box.

DINNER
- **Eat a light**, soupy, easily digestible meal at 6pm each evening (see pp.106–13).

Yoga and meditation

Practise neck exercises (pp.130–31) at work to take a break from the computer. Start doing yoga and meditation at the weekend, then introduce weekday sessions too.

- **10–30 minutes** of pranayama and asanas (see pp.122–59).
- **10 minutes** of meditation (see pp.176–77).

EASY CHANGES

These easy changes will have a noticeable affect on your health, providing added motivation for you to continue more challenging lifestyle practices.

- **Avoid sugary snacks** one day a week.
- **Replace sweets** with fresh or dried fruit.
- **Only drink hot** or warm Ayurvedic water during the day (see p.85).

ADVICE FOR VATA

Those of a vata nature should try to:

- **Perform a self-massage** with soothing oils – aim to give yourself two massages a week.
- **Introduce regularity** by eating your meals at the same time every day.

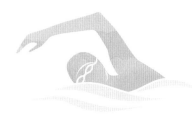

Physical exercise and activity

Doing regular exercise is the best way to build it into your routine. You may want to try out different types of exercise to see what you enjoy doing most.

- **If daily practice** is not possible, establish an exercise routine of 2–3 times a week.
- **Try to** do a form of exercise that suits your dominant dosha(s) (see pp.50–55).

The end of your day

Aim to go to sleep at 10pm or earlier by going to bed 30 minutes earlier each month. Then gradually build the following practices into your routine.

- **Finish any work** you need to do (both mentally and physically) an hour before going to bed, and reduce the presence of electronic devices from the room in which you sleep.
- **Do 5 minutes** of meditation (see pp.176–77) and yogic breathing exercises (see pp.124–27) before bed.

ADVICE FOR PITTA

Those of a pitta nature should try to:

- **Drink fewer alcoholic** drinks and reduce the amount of fried or spicy food you eat.
- **Perform alternate** nostril breathing every day (see pp.126–27).

ADVICE FOR KAPHA

Those of a kapha nature should try to:

- **Perform a self-massage** using kapha oils or herbal powder once a week (see pp.36–39).
- **Skip either** breakfast or dinner once a week if you are able to or arcn't hungry.

STEP
3

EXPANDING YOUR
HEALTHY LIFESTYLE

Now you have established a routine, you are ready to focus on how you can maintain it. You can also enhance your health and wellbeing further by diving deeper into what Ayurevda and yoga have to offer.

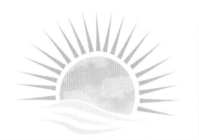

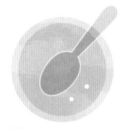

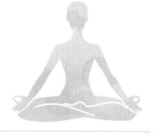

The start of your day

Get up at around 5.30am every morning. Then gradually add the following practices to your routine:

- **Do 30 minutes** of yoga and meditation each morning.
- **Give yourself** at least one self-massage each week (see pp.36–39).
- **Implement as much** of the hygiene routine on pp.34–35 as you are able to.

Food and mealtimes

Gradually build up the following practices until all of them become part of your lifestyle.

- **Eat your meals** at the same times each day.
- **Adapt your** meals to the seasons.
- **If inspired to,** try becoming a full vegetarian (see pp.64–67).
- **Identify which diet** suits the doshas in your body, and follow it if your dosha(s) are upset.
- **Start using** the spices that are best suited to your constitution and your palate.
- **Introduce** fasting on one day each week (see pp.86–87) if you are pitta or kapha, or half a day each week if you are vata.

Yoga and meditation

Do 1 hour of yoga and meditaton each day. This is best split into two 30-minute sessions, one in the morning, and another in the afternoon or evening.

- **Include both** breathing and relaxation exercises in your yoga sessions.
- **Go to a yoga class** at least once a week to benefit from the group energy and stay inspired.
- **Try going to a yoga retreat** once a year to fully recharge both physically and mentally. This will also give you motivation to stick with and deepen your practice.

"If you entertain healthy thoughts, you can keep good health."

SWAMI SIVANANDA

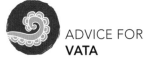

ADVICE FOR
VATA

Those of a vata nature should try to:

- **Eat warm** meals.
- **Try to have regular** bowel movements.
- **Perform regular** oil massages (see pp.36–39).

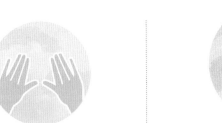 

Ayurvedic treatments

Always monitor the health of your agni and doshas (see pp.48–49). Try some of these practices:

- **Use basic home** remedies, such as only drinking Ayurvedic water (see p.85).
- **During the winter,** practise nasya up to three times a day (see pp.34–35).
- **If pitta** and kapha are strong in your constitution, do a long fast in the spring – for 2 days or up to a week (see pp.86–87).
- **Go to see an ayurvedic practitioner** for a panchakarma treatment, ideally during spring or autumn (see pp.194–95).

The end of your day

You should now be going to bed by 10pm each night. You could also try some of these suggestions.

- **Ban any computer** or phone screens from the room in which you sleep.
- **End each day** with enough time for soothing practices, such as quiet contemplation, meditation (see pp.180–81), or yogic breathing (see p.124–25).
- **Stop working** at least an hour before going to bed as often as you are able to.

ADVICE FOR
PITTA

Those of a pitta nature should try to:

- **Eat ghee** and milk.
- **Soothe their eyes** with rosewater or castor oil (see pp.34–35).
- **Be tolerant** to themselves and others.

ADVICE FOR
KAPHA

Those of a kapha nature should try to:

- **Limit their** intake of fatty and heavy foods.
- **Fast and** exercise on a regular basis.
- **Boost their** metabolism with a dry powder or kapha oil massage (see pp.36–39).

MAINTAINING
GOOD HEALTH

"Develop an inquisitive outlook towards the less obvious signs of ill health so as to keep from getting ill."

SWAMI SIVANANDA

HOW TO **RECOGNIZE PROBLEMS**

Disease starts to occur when the doshas are out of balance and/or agni is becoming weak. These boxes show symptoms that will help you recognize imbalances, and the following pages give advice on how to address these problems before more serious issues develop.

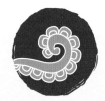

ELEVATED **VATA**

These symptoms can be signs that vata is starting to become irritated within the body and mind.

MENTAL
- **Lack of** concentration.
- **Sleeplessness.**
- **Sensitivity** (such as to noise and touch).
- **Exhaustion.**

PHYSICAL
- **Strong intolerance** to cold.
- **Restlessness and inability** to sit still.
- **Muscular tension.**
- **Constipation,** gas, or runny bowel movements.
- **Cravings for sweet,** salty, or sour food.
- **Stiffness or pain** in the joints.
- **Susceptibility** to common illnesses, such as colds or UTIs.

For information on lifestyle choices that you can make in order to treat elevated vata, move on to Pacifying vata, pp.50–51.

ELEVATED **PITTA**

These symptoms can be signs that pitta is starting to become irritated within the body and mind.

MENTAL
- **Irritation** or a short temper.
- **Prone to judge** others and themselves.
- **Overly competitive** behaviour.

PHYSICAL
- **Strong intolerance** for heat.
- **Burning sensations** (especially in the eyes).
- **A frequently red** and flushed face.
- **Sensitivity to** bright light.
- **Excessive thirst** or hunger.
- **Loose and** frequent bowel movements.
- **Increased sweating.**
- **Skin irritations.**
- **Cravings** for sweet and cold food and drink.
- **Heart burn** or sour eructation.

For information on lifestyle choices that you can make in order to treat elevated pitta, move on to Pacifying pitta, pp.52–53.

Responding to the body

The state of the body is in constant flux, with the strength of the doshas and the strength of agni always changing. It is helpful to develop an awareness of your body so that dosha imbalance and agni weakness can be noticed and addressed. Vata is the most easily elevated dosha due to its changing nature; it is also the quickest to rebalance. Pitta is more stable than vata, while kapha has the most stability – once kapha is increased it requires effort to bring it back into balance. The doshas that are most susceptible to imbalance for you will be those that are strongest in your constitution, or most influenced by your lifestyle (eg. kapha in a sedentary lifestyle), the season (eg. pitta in summer), or phase of your life (eg. vata in old age).

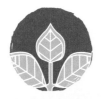

ELEVATED **KAPHA**

These symptoms can be signs that kapha is becoming irritated within the body and mind.

MENTAL

- **A lack** of inner drive and mental clarity.
- **Strong attachment** to things.

PHYSICAL

- **Excessively cold** skin.
- **Loss of** appetite and hunger.
- **Reduced sense** of taste and smell.
- **Weight gain.**
- **Feeling of heaviness** and sluggishness.
- **Fatigue** and lethargy.
- **Difficulty** becoming active.
- **Oily scalp** and dandruff.
- **Increased and** more viscous bodily secretions.
- **Sinusitis** or blocked sinuses.
- **Susceptibility** to colds with productive cough.

For information on lifestyle choices that you can make in order to treat elevated kapha, move on to Pacifying kapha, pp.54–55.

WEAK **AGNI**

These symptoms can be signs that your agni is weak and needs to be strengthened.

PHYSICAL

- **Indigestion.**
- **Fullness, heaviness,** or bloating after a meal.
- **Fatigue after** a normal meal.
- **Newly developed** food intolerances.
- **Reflux, heartburn,** or gastritis.
- **Undigested material** in your stool.

For information on lifestyle choices that you can make in order to treat a weak agni, move on to Strengthening agni, pp.56–57.

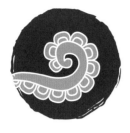

PACIFYING VATA

Vata is irregular, moving, light, dry, cool, fine, quick, and rough. It is pacified by practices that are regular, stable, heavy, oily, heating, viscous, slow, and smooth as these characteristics are opposite to its own.

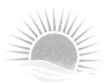

Lifestyle

Regularity is the key for pacifying vata. Those with a lot of vata have a tendency to become irregular in their movement and bodily rhythms, so try to keep to a fixed routine of eating, working, and sleeping.

WHAT TO DO

- **Maintain** a fixed daily routine.
- **Relax** regularly.
- **Go on** countryside walks in the sunshine.
- **Spend time** in quiet contemplation.
- **Listen to** calming music.
- **Take warm** baths.

WHAT NOT TO DO

- **Get too** stressed.
- **Eat at** irregular times.
- **Consume caffeine.**
- **Talk too** much.
- **Sleep too** little.
- **Exercise too** regularly.
- **Become exposed** to draughts and cold.
- **Activities that** cause sensory overload.

MASSAGE

Oil massage with heating oils is one of the best and most effective lifestyle practices to pacify elevated vata. If you have a tendency for vata imbalance, you should make oil massages a regular part of your routine. For more information about how to perform a self-massage and which oils to use for elevated vata, see pp.36–39.

EXERCISE

Grounding or strength-building exercise and any sport with slow, directed movements pacify vata. Weightlifting is particularly good as it provides stability and substance to counteract vata's lightness and mobilty. Those with a lot of vata in their constitution should be careful to avoid overexertion.

Diet

Those wishing to pacify vata benefit from a regular diet of warm, soupy food and only consuming drinks hot. A diet to pacify vata contains more fats and grains than diets for other doshas. For more information about a vata diet, see pp.72–75.

Yoga and meditation

Vata's tendency for movement, irregularity, and lightness benefits from the focus, quiet, and the calming and grounding effects of yoga and meditation. For more information, see chapter five on yoga (p.118) and chapter six on meditation (p.164).

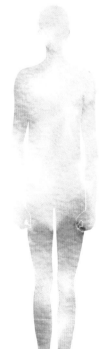

Practitioner treatments

You may wish to go to an Ayurvedic practitioner. They will assess you first, and may then recommend oil treatments, such as a full body massage or enemas to pacify vata (see pp.192–93), or a full panchakarma treatment to eliminate elevated vata (see pp.194–95).

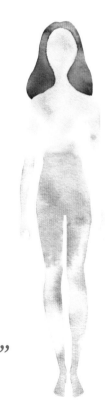

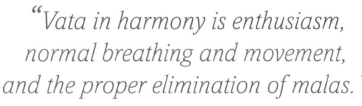

"Vata in harmony is enthusiasm, normal breathing and movement, and the proper elimination of malas."

CHARAKA

PACIFYING PITTA

Pitta is hot, liquid, sharp, light, quickly penetrating, sour, and slightly oily. It is pacified by practices that are cooling, soothing, heavy, slightly drying, and mild as these characteristics are opposite to its own.

Lifestyle

Those with a lot of pitta tend towards intensity both in their emotions and activities. They benefit from a mild and moderate work and personal life. Be sure to do soothing hobbies, and avoid activities that might provoke strong emotions.

WHAT TO DO

- **Oil massages** with cooling oils.
- **Go swimming.**
- **Go on walks** in the woods or in the shade, avoiding the sun.
- **Take cool baths.**
- **Listen to** calming music.

WHAT NOT TO DO

- **Sunbathe** or stay in the sun too long.
- **Get stressed.**
- **Use saunas** and steam rooms.
- **Give in** to strong anger or irritation.
- **Engage in** competitive activities.

MASSAGE

Pitta is pacified by cooling or soothing oils, such as coconut or almond oil, which counteract its heat and sharpness. For more information about how to perform a self massage and which oils to use for elevated pitta, see pp.36–39.

EXERCISE

Swimming and outdoor exercises in the shade are the best forms of exercise for pitta. Those with a lot of pitta will benefit from non-competitive sports, reigning in their competitiveness and focusing on enjoying the exercise.

Diet

Elevated pitta can be pacified by eating four times a day in small portions, avoiding pungent, sour foods, and adding cold, raw food to their diet. A diet to pacify pitta contains more vegetables than a vata diet, and more grains than a kapha diet. For more information about a pitta diet, see pp.76–79.

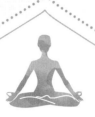

Yoga and meditation

The pitta drive and competitiveness are directed inward during yoga practice, developing body awareness rather than competitiveness. Meditaton then soothes the sharp pitta nature. For more information, see chapter five on yoga (p.118) and chapter six on meditation (p.164).

Practitioner treatments

You may wish to go to an Ayurvedic practitioner. They will assess you first, and may then recommend treatments such as an eye bath or a massage with cooling and soothing oils to pacify pitta (see pp.192–93), or a panchakarma treatment to eliminate elevated pitta (see pp.194–95).

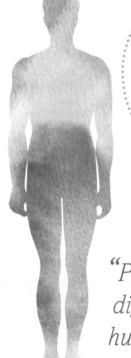

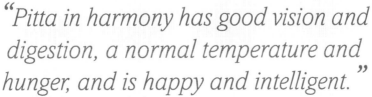

"Pitta in harmony has good vision and digestion, a normal temperature and hunger, and is happy and intelligent."

CHARAKA

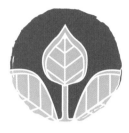

PACIFYING KAPHA

Kapha is cool, heavy, oily, stable, and soft. It is pacified by practices that are heating, light, dry, moving, and rough as these characteristics are opposite to its own.

Lifestyle

Those looking to pacify kapha should find ways that they can challenge themselves, be active, and change their routines every now and again. Stimulation is the key to counterbalance inertia and stability, which can eventually become rigidity.

WHAT TO DO

- **Dry-powder** or oil massages.
- **Take warm** baths.
- **Listen to** lively music.
- **Learn** new things.
- **Deviate** from your routine.
- **Seek out** stimulating company.

WHAT NOT TO DO

- **Be too** sedentary.
- **Sleep too** much.
- **Gain too** much weight.
- **Be exposed to** cold.
- **Live a** secluded lifestyle.

MASSAGE

Heating or stimulating massages, such as those using dry powder, silk gloves, or heating oils, pacify kapha. For more information about how to perform a self-massage and which oils to use for elevated kapha, see pp.36–39.

EXERCISE

Exercise is important for those with strong kapha as it stimulates their slower metabolism. Most benefit comes from the speed, activity, and competition provided by group sports. Dancing is also good as its lightness and movement balance kapha's heaviness and stability.

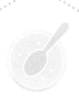

Diet

To pacify kapha, try to avoid overeating, or eating food that is too heavy. You might want to skip the occasional meal, fast regularly, and generally eat less. It is best to stick to warm meals and avoid heavy, greasy foods, or eating too many grains. For more information about a kapha diet, see pp.80–81.

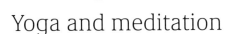

Yoga and meditation

The tendency for lethargy and inertia caused by kapha is eased by yoga's stimulation of prana (vital energy). The resulting sense of lightness and clarity is strengthened during meditation. For more information, see chapter five on yoga (p.118) and chapter six on meditation (p.164).

Practitioner treatments

You may wish to go to an Ayurvedic practitioner. They will assess you first, and may then recommend treatments such as herbal bolus or dry-powder massage to pacify kapha (see pp.192–93), or a panchakarma treatment to eliminate elevated kapha (see pp.194–95).

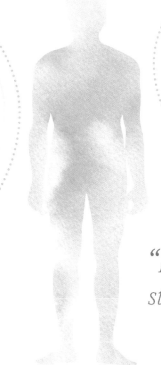

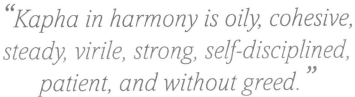

"Kapha in harmony is oily, cohesive, steady, virile, strong, self-disciplined, patient, and without greed."

CHARAKA

STRENGTHENING AGNI

Maintaining agni is one of the key principles of Ayurveda, and looking after our agni may now be one of our most important tasks, as it is weakened by most aspects of a modern lifestyle.

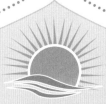

Lifestyle

Ayurveda teaches us how to keep agni strong and healthy, and how to restore its function if compromised. This revolves around what, how, and when we eat, as well as how regularly we exercise.

WHAT TO DO

- **Eat at the** same times each day.
- **Eat a light** and easily digestible diet of fresh, non-processed food.
- **Fast regularly** according to your health and dosha.
- **Drink hot** or warm water.
- **Exercise regularly.**

WHAT NOT TO DO

- **Overload your** stomach.
- **Eat when** you are not hungry.
- **Have cold** drinks.
- **Become stressed,** or eat a heavy diet during periods of stress.
- **Have too** sedentary a lifestyle.

MASSAGE

The agni in the tissues needs to be strong in order for massage oil to be digested. A full oil self-massage can be too much too digest if your agni is weak. Stimulating oils, or dry-powder or silk glove massages are a good alternative (see pp.36–39).

EXERCISE

Exercise stimulates and strengthens agni and the entire digestive process. Try to exercise every day, or at least two to three times a week.

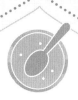

Diet

Those wishing to strengthen agni benefit from using plenty of spices in their food and fasting one day a week (see pp.86–87). Avoid eating too much, or foods that are too heavy. For more information about how to eat for strengthening agni, see pp.84–85.

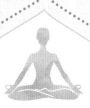

Yoga

Most yoga asanas have an agni-strengthening effect. A full yoga session will stimulate your metabolism and the agni in your digestive system, ensuring that you are ready to fully digest your meals. For more information, see chapter six on yoga (p.118)

Practitioner treatments

As well as the lifestyle and diet advice essential for strengthening agni, an Ayurvedic practitioner may recommend a course of therapeutic, agni-strengthening herbs, most of which also digest ama (see pp.196–97).

"The secret of being healthy and happy at all times is to be a little hungry all the time."

SWAMI SIVANANDA

FOOD, DIET,
AND RECIPES

*"Let your diet be anything, but it
should pass this test: it should protect
health and prevent disease."*

CHARAKA

THE **HEALING POWER** OF FOOD

Nutrition is called "the great medicine" in Ayurveda. A wholesome, well-balanced diet is the foundation of health, strength, and happiness, for both mind and body.

A healthy diet

The food you eat should be appetizing and appeal to all your senses. Make gradual changes to your diet by cutting down on unwholesome foods and introducing healthy ones in their place. With practice you will find the diet best suited to your taste and constitution.

A well-balanced diet consists of two-thirds nourishing foods, which help build tissue, and one-third purifying foods, which prevent kapha increase and excess tissue build-up (see p.26).

- **Nourishing foods:** grains, fruit, milk, dairy products, nuts, fats, and starchy vegetables, such as potatoes.
- **Purifying foods:** pulses and all other vegetables except those that are rajasic or tamasic (see p.65).

Drinking and eating

A small glass of hot water or water at room temperature half an hour before a meal and during a meal is beneficial. More than that will weaken agni. After a meal, wait at least one hour before having a drink, so as not to weaken agni or increase kapha.

ORIGIN

Regional foods that are fresh and ripe, rather than imported foods, are the best choice (see pp.66–67).

TIMING

The season, the time of day, and your phase of life all tell you which foods are best to eat. In winter, meals should be rich and nourishing; in summer, light and cooling. Make lunch your biggest meal.

QUALITY

Food should be organic, fresh, and selected according to its taste, heating or cooling quality, digestibility, and effect on the doshas and tissues. Avoid processed and pre-packaged foods and meals (see pp.66–67).

QUANTITY

Don't eat too much or too little. Fill your stomach half with solid food, one quarter with liquids and leave one quarter empty.

Follow the eight *guiding principles to ensure the food you eat has the power of healing.*

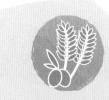

COMBINATION

The body's ability to digest is affected by how different foods are combined (see box, right).

PREPARATION

You are not what you eat, but what you digest. Naturally grown food that is properly prepared – ideally heated or cooked – is easiest to digest and absorb (see pp.88–89).

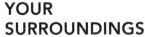

YOUR SURROUNDINGS

The atmosphere you cook and eat in, and the state of your kitchen play an important role (see pp.88–89). Work in a tidy, positive environment.

YOU

You, the person who eats, are important. The healthiest food can become poison if you are in a hurry, stressed, ill, or have a weak agni.

❌ INCOMPATIBLE FOODS

Some foods become hard to digest if eaten in large amounts at the wrong time, or together with certain other foods. They weaken agni, disturb the doshas, create blockage, and damage the tissues. Only people with a very strong agni, or who are used to eating these foods, will be able to digest them.

Try to avoid:

- **Milk with fruit,** fish, meat, yogurt, tomatoes, or pulses
- **Hot foods with** cold foods
- **Hot drinks** with honey, alcohol, or yogurt
- **Ghee and honey** combined in equal quantities
- **Cold foods** in winter.

"If you strive for bliss, your diet should be such that new disease cannot manifest and existing disease is alleviated."

CHARAKA

SIX TASTES

In Ayurveda every food or substance has at least one of the six tastes: sweet, sour, salty, pungent, bitter, and astringent. To properly satisfy the body and mind, a full meal should include all six tastes.

Effect on doshas

The six tastes all have different qualities, such as cooling or oily. Each taste has an effect on the doshas, because they come from the same elements as the doshas and share the same qualities. A taste that has the same quality as a dosha will increase it. To pacify a dosha that is elevated in your constitution, emphasize tastes with the opposite qualities in your meal.

Three phases of digestion

An Ayurvedic meal starts with the sweet kapha phase, when the elements water and earth are digested. Ideally, foods with a sweet taste (such as grains, and also dessert) should be eaten first as they need a strong agni. This may be new to the Western palate, but it is well worth a try.

Then comes the sour pitta phase, which digests the element fire. Eat sour and salty foods next. These support agni.

Finally, there is the vata phase, which digests air and ether. Consume bitter and astringent foods last. These support the vata phase and reduce kapha.

Follow the order of the tastes when eating your meal, starting with sweet and ending with astringent.

Cooling, heavy, oily

Water
Earth

1 SWEET
Sweet foods include: grains, ghee, pasta, bread, sugar, milk, cheese, potatoes, carrots, beetroot, squash, parsnips, cucumber, most fruits.

Heating, oily, and light

2 SOUR
Sour foods include: lemon, curd, buttermilk, tomatoes, tamarind, sour apples. Serve a slice of lemon and/or some yogurt with salt with your main meal.

Earth
Fire

3 SALTY
Salty foods include: tamari and soy sauce, and rock and sea salt.

Heating and oily

Water
Fire

Each taste is made up of two elements and has a unique combination of qualities. Each food has at least one taste, and many have two or more; for example, celery (bitter, pungent, salty).

"The tastes sour and pungent stimulate agni; the tastes bitter and astringent reduce tissue."

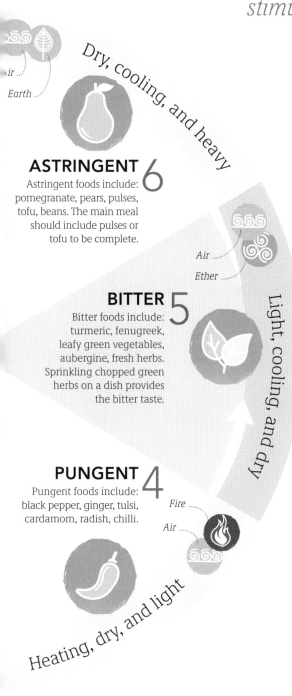

Dry, cooling, and heavy

ASTRINGENT 6
Astringent foods include:
pomegranate, pears, pulses,
tofu, beans. The main meal
should include pulses or
tofu to be complete.

BITTER 5
Bitter foods include:
turmeric, fenugreek,
leafy green vegetables,
aubergine, fresh herbs.
Sprinkling chopped green
herbs on a dish provides
the bitter taste.

PUNGENT 4
Pungent foods include:
black pepper, ginger, tulsi,
cardamom, radish, chilli.

ir

Earth

Air

Ether

Fire

Air

Light, cooling, and dry

Heating, dry, and light

EFFECT ON VATA
Vata is made from
ether and air.

Sweet, sour, salty tastes
pacify vata.

Pungent, bitter, astringent
tastes increase vata.

EFFECT ON PITTA
Pitta is made from fire
and water.

Sweet, bitter, astringent
tastes pacify pitta.

Pungent, salty, sour tastes
increase pitta.

EFFECT ON KAPHA
Kapha is made from
earth and water.

Pungent, bitter, astringent
tastes pacify kapha.

Sweet, sour, salty tastes
increase kapha.

SATTVIC DIET

Sattva is the energy of harmony and clarity. A sattvic diet helps create happiness of mind and is made up of pure foods that are delicious, wholesome, and give mental strength.

Energy and joy

Sattva is one of the three energies of the mind, or gunas (see pp.166–67). A sattvic diet consists of pure foods that give health, energy, joy, peace, and clarity. Our mind and body are strongly influenced by what we eat and drink. As you start to follow a sattvic diet, the positive experience of sattva will lead you to want to refine your tastes and food choices further.

A sattvic meal is prepared from fresh, natural ingredients. It is eaten freshly cooked and in moderate amounts, sitting down, and taking your time. It is easy to digest and leaves you feeling light and energized.

The guidelines opposite are designed to help you make conscious decisions about your diet. Remember that changes should be made gradually, but consistently.

> *"The foods which increase purity, strength, health, and joy are sattvic."*
>
> BHAGAVAD GĪTĀ

SATTVIC FOODS

Include as many of the following in your diet as possible:

 Whole grains, such as barley, millet, wheat, oats, unpolished rice, and quinoa

 Fresh vegetables – green leafy vegetables, and seeded vegetables, such as cucumber and squash

 Ripe, fresh fruits, such as pears, apples, plums, peaches, apricots, mangos, figs, and avocados

 Nuts, seeds, and legumes, such as mung dhal, lentils, chana dhal, chickpeas, cashews, almonds, sunflower seeds, and pumpkin seeds

 Dairy products – organic, fresh milk, ghee, fresh cheese, curd, and yogurt from happy cows or goats

 Spices that are not too stimulating: coriander, pepper, turmeric, cumin, parsley, and rock salt in moderation

 Natural sweeteners, such as jaggery, honey, molasses, and maple or agave syrup.

HEALTHY SWAPS

To achieve a sattvic diet, try replacing the foods on the top line, in red, with their alternatives below, in green.

MEAT, FISH, AND **POULTRY** AS A PROTEIN SOURCE	**EGGS** AS A BINDER OR PROTEIN SOURCE	**EGGS** AS A RAISING AGENT	ONIONS	VINEGAR
PULSES, TOFU, OR TEMPEH	CHICKPEA FLOUR, TOFU, AND **TAPIOCA** STARCH	BAKING POWDER OR YOGURT PLUS SPARKLING WATER	GINGER OR CELERY	LEMON JUICE

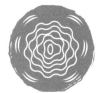

RAJASIC FOODS

Rajas is the energy of agitation (see p.167). Rajasic foods increase negative emotions, such as lust, anger, greed, selfishness, violence, and egoism. Rajasic foods are excessively pungent, bitter, sour, salty, dry, and burning. Tobacco is rajasic, and sattvic food eaten in a hurry becomes rajasic.

Try to avoid the following, which are rajasic:
- Unripe fruit
- Highly pungent spices, such as chilli, in excess
- Caffeine (in coffee, black and green tea, and soft drinks)
- Too many sweets
- Onions
- Garlic
- Radishes
- Hard cheese
- Eggs
- Refined (white) sugar
- Soft drinks
- Prepared mustards
- Heavily spiced and salted convenience foods
- Snacks with artificial additives
- Stimulants of all kinds.

TAMASIC FOODS

Tamas is the energy of resistance (see p.167). Tamasic foods are stale, decomposed, or unclean and can make you dull, inert, lazy, and depressed. Meat, poultry, fish, and all intoxicants (such as alcohol, marijuana, and opium) are all tamasic in nature. Sattvic food taken in excessive quantity (overeating) becomes tamasic.

Try to avoid the following, which are tamasic:
- Overripe fruit
- Mushrooms
- Vinegar
- Peanuts
- Meat
- Poultry
- Fish
- Fermented foods
- Food that has been burnt
- Fried or deep-fried foods
- Barbecued food
- Reheated meals
- Canned food
- Processed food
- Pre-prepared meals
- Leftovers.

CONSIDER **VEGETARIANISM**

The yogic diet is based on sattvic foods, which means it is lacto-vegetarian. There are many benefits that come with eating only vegetarian food.

Why be a vegetarian?

Maintaining a happy and healthy mind and body relies on eating fresh, nourishing food. A well-balanced vegetarian diet consisting of grains, vegetables, fruit, herbs, milk, ghee, and vegetable oils provides all the nourishment required. Vegetarianism has a positive impact on both the health of the individual and the world (see right).

Choose wisely

Fresh, ripe foods are the best choices for a sattvic diet. Try to avoid tinned food and frozen food. Meals should be freshly prepared, not processed.

Wherever possible, aim to:

- **Shop organic** – choose foods grown in fertile soil free from pesticides
- **Shop local** – farmers' markets and home-grown produce are ideal
- **Avoid supermarket produce** that has been prepackaged and imported.

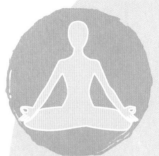

TO INCREASE **SATTVA**

To increase sattva (see pp.166–67), and enhance spiritual growth. Meat, poultry, fish, and eggs are considered rajasic and tamasic.

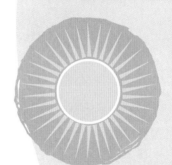

FOR **NOURISHMENT**

The further away from the original source of energy – the sun – your food is, the less nourishing it is. Plant-based foods are lighter and easier to digest than meat, which is a burden on the digestive tract.

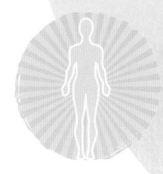

FOR GOOD **HEALTH**

According to scientific evidence, those with a balanced vegetarian diet have fewer chronic diseases – most notably, they have lower cholesterol, are less obese, and have a lower risk of heart disease.

"May you all attain perfect health, longevity, and peace by living on a vegetarian diet, which is helpful for meditation and healthy living."

SWAMI SIVANANDA

THROUGH
COMPASSION

Compassion, or non-violence, towards all living beings is an important part of Ayurveda (see pp.174–75). This includes animals.

TO FEED
THE WORLD

The growing human population is putting pressure on the planet's resources. The Earth can provide enough food for everyone – if we all eat a vegetarian diet.

TO PROTECT
THE EARTH

A vegetarian diet reduces the negative environmental impact of meat production, such as greenhouse gas emissions, water wastage, and water pollution.

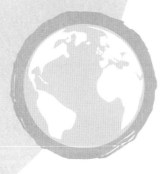

MODERN FOOD
PRODUCTION

Milk and butter contain the impressions of the animals they come from: the quality of their feed and their living conditions. Invest in the best you can afford.

High-quality products come from animals that enjoy the following living conditions:

- **A natural habitat**
- **Space to move**
- **Good-quality feed**
- **Freedom to choose** to eat those foods they need
- **No hormone** or antibiotic treatments
- **Freedom from** negative experiences, such as fear and stress.

These are six reasons *to consider changing to a vegetarian diet, which has both personal and global benefits.*

HERBS AND SPICES

According to Ayurveda, herbs and spices stimulate appetite, strengthen agni, and have beneficial therapeutic actions. To pacify an elevated dosha, make use of the herbs or spices that show a down arrow in the relevant column in the chart.

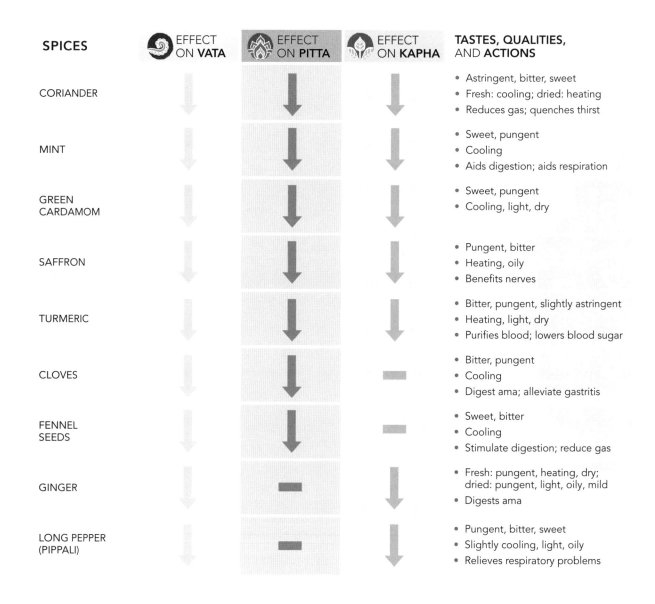

SPICES	EFFECT ON VATA	EFFECT ON PITTA	EFFECT ON KAPHA	TASTES, QUALITIES, AND ACTIONS
CORIANDER	↓	↓	↓	• Astringent, bitter, sweet • Fresh: cooling; dried: heating • Reduces gas; quenches thirst
MINT	↓	↓	↓	• Sweet, pungent • Cooling • Aids digestion; aids respiration
GREEN CARDAMOM	↓	↓	↓	• Sweet, pungent • Cooling, light, dry
SAFFRON	↓	↓	↓	• Pungent, bitter • Heating, oily • Benefits nerves
TURMERIC	↓	↓	↓	• Bitter, pungent, slightly astringent • Heating, light, dry • Purifies blood; lowers blood sugar
CLOVES	↓	↓	—	• Bitter, pungent • Cooling • Digest ama; alleviate gastritis
FENNEL SEEDS	↓	↓	—	• Sweet, bitter • Cooling • Stimulate digestion; reduce gas
GINGER	↓	—	↓	• Fresh: pungent, heating, dry; dried: pungent, light, oily, mild • Digests ama
LONG PEPPER (PIPPALI)	↓	—	↓	• Pungent, bitter, sweet • Slightly cooling, light, oily • Relieves respiratory problems

SPICES	EFFECT ON VATA	EFFECT ON PITTA	EFFECT ON KAPHA	TASTES, QUALITIES, AND ACTIONS
BASIL	↓	↑	↓	• Pungent, bitter • Heating • Fresh: decongestant
BAY LEAVES	↓	↑	↓	• Pungent, bitter • Heating • Reduce gas from pulses
CINNAMON	↓	↑	↓	• Pungent, bitter, sweet • Heating, light, dry • Digests ama; reduces gas
CUMIN	↓	↑	↓	• Pungent, sweet • Heating, light, dry • Stimulates appetite; reduces gas
FENUGREEK	↓	↑	↓	• Bitter • Heating • Reduces gastric hyperacidity
MUSTARD SEEDS	↓	↑	↓	• Pungent, bitter • Heating, dry • Digest ama
NUTMEG	↓	↑	↓	• Pungent, bitter, astringent • Heating • Aids sleep, aromatic
OREGANO	↓	↑	↓	• Bitter • Heating, dry • Digests ama; reduces gas
PARSLEY	↓	↑	↓	• Pungent, bitter • Light, dry, heating • Diuretic; digestive tonic
ROSEMARY	↓	↑	↓	• Pungent, bitter, astringent • Heating • Decongestant
CURRY LEAVES	↑	↓	↓	• Bitter, pungent • Heavy, dry, heating • Digestive tonic
CHILLI	↓	↑	↓	• Pungent • Heating, light, dry • Digests ama; lowers cholesterol

GHEE, SUGAR, AND **HONEY**

In Ayurveda, food is medicine. As well as being everyday ingredients, ghee, sugar, and honey have powerful healing properties. Ghee and honey strengthen agni (digestive fire) when taken in moderation.

Reaping the benefits

Sugar is the sweetener of choice in Ayurvedic cuisine. Honey is regarded as medicine. Both substances should be consumed in moderation.

The best forms of sugar to use are jaggery (unrefined cane sugar), which is available from some supermarkets, or sharkara (purified cane sugar), which can be found in specialist stores or online. Sharkara should not be confused with industrialized, refined white sugar, which has a similar appearance.

Ghee has a sweet taste. It rejuvenates the whole system and is a general tonic. If you are in good health, try to cook with ghee daily.

IMPORTANT NOTE

Avoid heating honey or taking it with hot substances, because according to Ayurveda, when honey is heated it produces ama, which acts as a toxin (see p.26). Honey should not be taken together with an equal quantity of ghee as this is also detrimental to health.

GHEE

Ghee is clarified butter, and is one of the best fats to use for cooking. It is made by heating butter until all the water has evaporated and then filtering the milk solids until only the fat remains. For therapeutic purposes, the older the ghee is, the better its healing properties will be. It is said that ghee that is one hundred years old can even reduce kapha.

BENEFITS

Ghee has healing properties and improves mental function, the complexion, voice, eyes, and reproductive tissue. It is also used as a carrier for healing herbs, and is added to some herbal oils. Here are just a few examples of the medicinal uses of ghee:

- **Soothing burns**
- **Aiding in** wound healing
- **As a brain tonic**
- **Purifying the blood,** and treating skin diseases
- **Soothing and purifying** the eyes.

QUALITIES

- **Heavy**
- **Soft**
- **Oily**
- **Cooling**

EFFECT ON THE DOSHAS

Pacifies vata and pitta. Increases kapha.

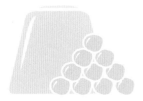

SUGAR

Jaggery and sharkara are the two most commonly used forms of sugar in Ayurvedic cuisine. Jaggery is thickened and solidified cane sugar syrup and contains many bioactive phytochemicals. It is available in lumps or as a powder. Sharkara is white sugar, which has been carefully purified. Compared to refined white sugar (which is heating), sharkara is cooling, lighter, and easier to digest.

BENEFITS

Opt for older jaggery wherever possible, as it is easier to digest than fresh jaggery, which increases kapha and can lead to asthma.

Sharkara only mildly increases kapha. It has the following benefits:

- **Diuretic**
- **Purifies** the blood
- **Soothes burning** sensations
- **Quenches** thirst
- **Beneficial for** the eyes.

QUALITIES

- **Heavy**
- **Moisturizing**
- **Cold**

EFFECT ON THE DOSHAS

Pacifies vata and pitta. Increases kapha.

HONEY

Honey's astringent, subtle, and dry qualities make it the ideal substance for reducing kapha. The best variety is honeydew honey (also known as forest honey), which is penetrating and sharp. Those with a lot of pitta or vata should consume honey in moderation. As it is a desiccant, honeydew honey can reduce body weight, in conjunction with a suitable diet for weight loss.

BENEFITS

Honey improves the skin, bones, nerves, eyes, heart, and voice and is an antimicrobial. It also has the following specific uses:

- **Treating coughs** and sore throats
- **Treating burns** (used externally)
- **Helping wounds** to heal (used externally)
- **As a carrier** for many herbal medicines to improve their absorption and enhance their effect
- **Honey that is more than** one year old reduces body fat. (Fresh honey increases body weight.)

QUALITIES

- **Cooling**
- **Astringent**
- **Subtle**
- **Dry**

EFFECT ON THE DOSHAS

Increases vata and pitta. Pacifies kapha.

THE **VATA DIET**

A vata diet is suitable for anyone who needs to pacify and reduce vata, whether or not vata is one of the dominant doshas in their constitution. It is nourishing, tissue-building, and gives strength and vitality.

Understanding a vata diet

If vata is one of your dominant doshas and your doshas are in balance, you do not need to follow a special vata diet. You should aim to eat a balanced diet containing all the six tastes.

Eating for vata

If you need to follow a special vata diet (see right), you will benefit from eating warm foods. Meals that are both warm and soupy and that contain high-quality fats are easily digested and drive out gas. A warm meal supports agni and a soupy, oily meal gives strength and nourishes the sense organs.

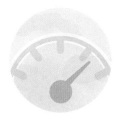

When to follow a vata diet

You should follow a vata diet if:

- **You have elevated vata**
- **You feel your vata** may become elevated as a result of your lifestyle, or because you have a lot of vata in your constitution
- **In dry, windy,** and cold weather
- **During late autumn** and winter
- **When you are** in a region that aggravates vata, such as high-altitude mountains
- **In old age,** when vata is high.

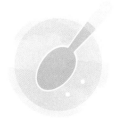

What and how to eat

The way you eat and how you prepare your food are important. Select foods with opposite qualities and tastes to cool, dry, irregular vata.

These are the most important aspects of the vata diet:

- **Qualities:** hot, liquid, oily, heavy
- **Tastes:** sweet, sour, salty
- **Regular meals**
- **Eating in a calm** and unhurried atmosphere
- **Warm, cooked foods,** preferably soups
- **Drinking hot** beverages only.

"Food should be taken in a calm and quiet place, free from anxiety and sorrow, observing silence."

SWAMI SIVANANDA

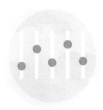

Adapting your meals

Compared to the other doshas, vata benefits from a diet that includes increased amounts of the following tastes, textures, and qualities:

- **Sweet tastes,** in the form of carbohydrates
- **Liquids, in the form** of soupy foods and sauces
- **Oiliness, from** dairy products, and fats in the form of ghee or most vegetable oils (see p.75)
- **Salty or sweet** chutneys added to your meal.

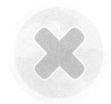

What to avoid

If you are following a vata diet you should reduce or avoid:

- **Qualities:** cold, dry, light
- **Tastes:** pungent, bitter, astringent
- **Fasting** – if you have a lot of vata in your constitution, you should not fast for longer than 16 hours; if you have elevated vata, you should not fast at all
- **Irregular meals**
- **Eating on the go**
- **Eating when under stress**
- **Raw, cold, and dry foods**, such as salad
- **Cold drinks.**

Agni and vata

Elevated vata weakens agni. If you are following a vata diet, remember to take good care of agni. Follow the guidelines on pp.84–85, and try the following:

- **One or two slices** of fresh ginger with a pinch of rock salt and lemon juice before meals
- **Curd or yogurt** with a pinch of salt taken with your meal.

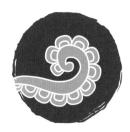

FOODS FOR **VATA**

If it is appropriate for you to follow a vata diet (see pp.72–73), use these pages to discover the foods to choose and the foods to avoid.

Balancing vata

The pie chart (see right) shows the proportions of different foods to eat for a vata diet as part of your daily meals. Specific ingredients that are ideal for pacifying vata are given around the outside of the chart.

FOODS TO **REDUCE OR AVOID**

Soothe vata by reducing or avoiding:

- **Grains:** millet, brown rice, any wholemeal grain, corn, barley, buckwheat, oat bran, cold cereals, puffed cereals, crispbread, cereal flakes, rice flakes, puffed rice or corn cakes, popcorn
- **Vegetables:** all types of cabbage: kale, Brussels sprouts, kohlrabi, broccoli, cauliflower
- **Pulses:** chickpeas, aduki beans, white beans, black beans
- **Dairy products:** sheep's milk cheese, buffalo mozzarella
- **Nuts and seeds:** bitter almonds
- **Spices and herbs:** chilli, cayenne pepper
- **Drinks:** cold or caffeinated beverages: coffee, black tea, green tea, and fruit or vegetable juice in cold weather
- **Fruit:** astringent fruit: pears, unripe bananas.

55% GRAINS

Grains
Wheat, white rice, spelt, quinoa, cooked oats, yeast-free bread.

Vegetables
Fennel, cucumber, carrots, squash, okra, parsnip, beetroot, spinach, asparagus, sweet potatoes, courgettes, sweet peas, cooked and peeled tomatoes*, artichokes*.

Additional items

Add flavour to your meals with spices, herbs, sweeteners, and salt. Fresh fruit should be eaten outside of meal times. Take drinks before or during your meal, not immediately after (wait one hour).

SPICES AND HERBS
These include: aniseed, basil, dill, fennel, ginger, cinnamon, cardamom, cumin, turmeric, bay leaves, cloves, sage, marjoram, rosemary.

20%
VEGETABLES

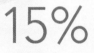

Fats
Ghee, all cooking oils except for coconut oil.

SALT
The salty taste pacifies vata. Opt for local or Himalayan rock salt (rose-coloured or white).

15%
FATS, DAIRY PRODUCTS, NUTS, SEEDS

Dairy products
Salted buttermilk, salted butter, fresh cheese, heated cows' milk, mozzarella, sour and sweet cream, hard cheese*.

SWEETENERS
Small quantities of: raw cane sugar, jaggery, fruit juice concentrate, molasses, honey.*

FRUIT
Sweet and/or sour fruit, for example: grapes, pineapple, apples, avocados, fresh dates, strawberries, figs, oranges, kiwis, limes.

10%
PULSES

Nuts and seeds
Nuts roasted in ghee or soaked in water for three hours and peeled. Almonds, walnuts, hazelnuts, pumpkin seeds, sunflower seeds, sesame seeds.

DRINKS
Juices: apple, berry, mango, orange. Lemon juice with rock salt. Teas: fennel, chamomile, lemon balm.

Pulses
Mung beans, kidney beans, soy milk, red lentils*, soy products*.

Foods that are marked with an asterisk *will pacify the vata dosha if taken in small amounts – consume in moderation.*

THE **PITTA DIET**

A pitta diet is suitable for anyone who needs to pacify and reduce pitta, whether or not pitta is one of the dominant doshas in their constitution. It aims to purify the blood, and reduce heat and sourness in the body.

Understanding a pitta diet

If pitta is one of your dominant doshas and your doshas are in balance, you do not need to follow a special pitta diet. You should aim to eat a balanced diet containing all the six tastes.

Eating for pitta

If you need to follow a special pitta diet (see right), you will benefit from eating plenty of vegetables, fruit, and carbohydrates, a good amount of protein, and not too much fat. Healthy pitta is the only one of the three doshas that benefits from raw foods, such as salad.

When to follow a pitta diet

You should follow a pitta diet if:

- **You have elevated pitta**
- **You feel your pitta** may become elevated as a result of your lifestyle, or because you have a lot of pitta in your constitution
- **During the summer** and early autumn, and in hot and humid weather, when pitta is high
- **When you are** in regions that aggravate pitta, such as the tropics.

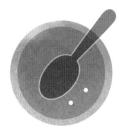

What and how to eat

The way you eat and how you prepare your food is important. To pacify pitta, select foods with opposite qualities and tastes to hot, liquid, and light. Be careful, however, not to eat too many cold and heavy foods, which compromise agni. These are the most important aspects of the pitta diet:

- **Qualities:** dry, mild, warm or cool, slightly heavy
- **Tastes:** sweet, bitter, astringent
- **Regular meals**
- **Eating in a** friendly atmosphere
- **Plenty of** fruit and vegetables
- **Eating four small meals a day** or three meals a day and an afternoon snack of sweet fruit.

"Do not eat when you are angry. Rest for a while until the mind becomes calm and then take your food."

SWAMI SIVANANDA

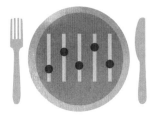

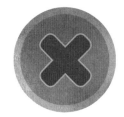

Adapting your meals

As part of your pitta diet, make simple changes to your meals that will help to pacify pitta. Try adding the following to your usual dishes:

- **Ghee** (in moderate quantities)
- **Fresh herbs** that are bitter and cooling, such as coriander and mint
- **Green cardamom** in moderation – it is cooling but also pungent
- **Rosewater,** which is cooling
- **Coconut milk or oil,** which is cooling.

What to avoid

If you are following a pitta diet you should reduce or avoid:

- **Qualities:** hot, light, oily
- **Tastes:** pungent, salty, sour
- **Fried food**
- **Foods that** are too hot
- **Hot or pungent** teas
- **Eating when** angry or irritated
- **Eating in** a hurry
- **Having heated** conversations during a meal
- **Skipping too** many meals.

Agni and pitta

Even though pitta and agni share the element of fire, an elevated pitta does not necessarily mean a healthy digestive fire; in fact, often, the opposite.

If you have an irritated or elevated pitta, take care of agni with:

- **Bitter foods**
- **Physical exercise**
- **Herbs and spices** – cook with long pepper (pippali), cloves, cardamom, and mint.

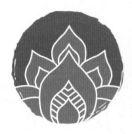

FOODS FOR **PITTA**

If it is appropriate for you to follow a pitta diet (see pp.76–77), use these pages to discover the foods to choose and the foods to avoid.

Balancing pitta

The pie chart (see right) shows the proportions of different foods to eat for a pitta diet as part of your daily meals. Specific ingredients that are ideal for pacifying pitta are given around the outside of the chart.

FOODS TO **REDUCE OR AVOID**

Soothe pitta by reducing or avoiding:

- **Grains:** rye
- **Vegetables:** radishes, seaweed, hot peppers, raw tomatoes
- **Dairy products:** yogurt, hard, spicy cheese, gorgonzola, Parmesan, kefir, sour cream
- **Fats:** sesame oil, mustard seed oil
- **Nuts and seeds:** cashews, peanuts, hazelnuts, unpeeled almonds, brazil nuts, pine nuts, pistachios, walnuts
- **Spices and herbs:** chilli and cayenne pepper, mustard seeds, black pepper
- **Drinks:** orange juice, tomato juice, alcohol, coffee
- **Sweeteners:** white sugar, honeydew honey, chocolate
- **Fruit:** cranberries, strawberries, rhubarb, redcurrants, blackcurrants, sour cherries.

50%
GRAINS

*Foods that are marked with an asterisk *will pacify the pitta dosha if taken in small amounts – consume in moderation.*

Grains
Amaranth, wholemeal grains, Basmati rice, spelt, barley, oats, quinoa, wheat, wheat bran, corn*.

25%
VEGETABLES

15%
PULSES

10%
FATS
DAIRY PRODUCTS
NUTS
SEEDS

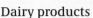

Vegetables
Artichokes, aubergines (baked or grilled and peeled), green leafy vegetables, cauliflower, broccoli, cucumber, kohlrabi, all types of cabbage, peas, carrots, potatoes, squash, okra, green bell pepper, parsnips, beetroot, salad, celeriac, asparagus, sweet potatoes, cooked, peeled, and seedless tomatoes*.

Pulses
Pitta can eat all pulses. Eat soaked and cooked well with plenty of spices. Try: aduki beans, chickpeas, yellow and red lentils, soy products, mung beans, kidney beans.

Fats
Ghee is best. Oils: coconut, olive, canola, linseed, sunflower.

Dairy products
Buttermilk, unsalted butter, fresh cheese, watered down cows' milk mozzarella, sweet cream, unsalted soft goats' cheese, mild, soft, low-fat cheese.

Nuts and seeds
Coconut, almonds soaked in water for three hours and peeled, sunflower seeds, coconut milk, almond milk.

Additional items

Add flavour to your meals with spices, herbs, sweeteners, and salt. Fresh fruit should be eaten outside of meal times. Take drinks before or during your meal, not immediately after (wait one hour).

SPICES AND HERBS
These include: basil, curry leaves, fenugreek, fennel, coriander, cardamom, cumin, turmeric, mint, peppermint, sage, long pepper, rosewater.

SALT
To pacify pitta, eat fewer salty foods. Opt for local or Himalayan rock salt (rose-coloured or white).

SWEETENERS
Small quantities of: maple syrup, raw cane sugar, juice concentrate, molasses, fresh honey.

FRUIT
Sweet and cooling fruit, for example: red grapes, sweet apples, apricots, avocados, bananas, blueberries, pears, dates, figs, plums, raisins.

DRINKS
Juices: apple, apricot, pear, vegetable, mango, pomegranate, sweet cherry. Teas: fennel, rosehip, jasmine, liquorice. Milk: almond milk, rice milk.

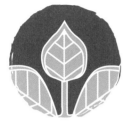

THE **KAPHA DIET**

A kapha diet is suitable for anyone who needs to pacify and reduce kapha, whether or not kapha is a dominant dosha in their constitution. It reduces excess tissue, opens blockages, and stimulates the metabolism.

Understanding a kapha diet

If kapha is one of your dominant doshas and your doshas are in balance, you do not need to follow a special kapha diet. You should aim to eat a balanced diet containing all the six tastes.

Eating for kapha

If you need to follow a special kapha diet (see right), you should try to keep your food intake light. The way you eat is more important than what you eat. Any heavy substance becomes light when eaten in small amounts, and any light substance becomes heavy when consumed in large amounts. Fast, eat less, and skip meals (see pp.86–87).

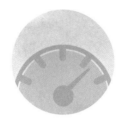

When to follow a kapha diet

You should follow a kapha diet if:

- **You have elevated kapha**
- **You feel your** kapha may become elevated as a result of your lifestyle, or because you have a lot of kapha in your constitution
- **During spring,** and if agni is weak then also during the cold and wet season, when kapha is high
- **When you are** in regions that elevate kapha, such as regions that have long winters, lots of ice and snow, or lots of rain and cold.

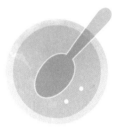

What and how to eat

The way you eat and how you prepare your food is important. Select foods with opposite qualities and tastes to cold, oily, heavy kapha. These are the most important aspects of the kapha diet:

- **Qualities:** hot, dry, light
- **Tastes:** pungent, bitter, astringent
- **Regular, warm meals** in good, lively company
- **Fasting or** reducing meals to two a day by skipping breakfast or dinner
- **Drinking hot** beverages only, and not drinking too much – a maximum of 1.5 litres per day.

"Simple and nourishing foods, moderation, and regular exercise go a long way to the attainment of health and longevity."

SWAMI SIVANANDA

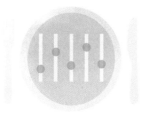

Adapting your meals

If you have a kapha constitution and are following a kapha diet to reduce kapha you will benefit from the following:

- **Eating plenty** of vegetables
- **Increased pulses** in your diet
- **Preparing food** using pungent spices or spice mixes, for example: ginger, pepper, a small amount of chilli or radish, or a spicy chutney
- **Dry foods.**

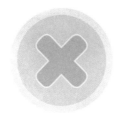

What to avoid

If you are following a kapha diet you should reduce or avoid:

- **All heavy,** cold, and oily foods
- **Cold and** heavy drinks
- **Tastes:** sweet, sour, salty
- **Milk and** milk products
- **Overeating**
- **Snacking**
- **Eating late** at night
- **Eating on** your own.

Agni and kapha

For kapha, a warm meal stimulates agni, tastes good, and is quickly digested. To keep agni strong, follow the guidelines on pp.84–85 and also try the following:

- **Bitter foods**
- **Physical exercise**
- **Cooking with ginger,** black pepper, a little chilli, and plenty of bitter spices, such as curry leaves, turmeric, and fenugreek seeds or leaves.

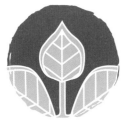

FOODS FOR **KAPHA**

If it is appropriate for you to follow a kapha diet (see pp.80–81), use these pages to discover the foods to choose and the foods to avoid.

Balancing kapha

The pie chart (see right) shows the proportions of different foods to eat for a kapha diet as part of your daily meals. Specific ingredients that are ideal for pacifying kapha are given around the outside of the chart.

FOODS TO **REDUCE** OR **AVOID**

Soothe kapha by reducing or avoiding:

- **Grains:** white flour, wheat
- **Vegetables:** avocados, cucumbers, pumpkins/squash, tomatoes, sweet potatoes
- **Pulses:** kapha can eat all pulses, as they are astringent
- **Dairy products:** all dairy products not listed opposite
- **Nuts and seeds:** all nuts and seeds not listed opposite
- **Spices and herbs:** kapha should reduce salt
- **Drinks:** cold drinks. Fruit juice needs to be watered down
- **Sweeteners:** white sugar
- **Fruit:** avocados, bananas, dates, fresh figs, honeydew melon, cherries, mangoes, watermelon, grapes.

45%
GRAINS

Grains
Millet, corn, buckwheat, brown rice, rye, whole wheat, amaranth, barley, quinoa, puffed rice or corn cakes, cereal flakes, popcorn, bran, white rice*, spelt*, rolled oats*, corn*.

30%
VEGETABLES

15%
PULSES

10%
FATS
DAIRY PRODUCTS
NUTS
SEEDS

Vegetables
Artichokes, aubergines (baked or grilled and peeled), green leafy vegetables, such as spinach, green beans, cauliflower, broccoli, kale, leek, okra, bell peppers, spicy peppers, radishes, all types of cabbage, peas, potatoes, squash, okra, parsnips, beetroot, celeriac, asparagus.

Pulses
Eat soaked and cooked well with plenty of spices. Aduki beans, peas, chickpeas, yellow and red lentils, mung beans, kidney beans, soy milk*, soy beans*, tofu*, seitan*.

Fats
Olive oil, canola oil, mustard oil (a maximum of 2 tablespoons per day).

Dairy products
Buttermilk, cottage cheese, skimmed goats' milk*, unsalted goats' cheese with spices*

Nuts and seeds
Pumpkin seeds*, sunflower seeds*, linseeds*.

*Foods that are marked with an asterisk *will pacify the kapha dosha if taken in small amounts – consume in moderation.*

Additional items

Add flavour to your meals with spices, herbs, sweeteners, and salt. Fresh fruit should be eaten outside of meal times. Take drinks before or during your meal, not immediately after (wait one hour).

SPICES AND HERBS
These include: anise, fenugreek, cayenne, chilli, parsley, marjoram, nutmeg, mustard seeds, coriander.

SALT
Be moderate with your use of salt. Opt for small amounts of local or Himalayan rock salt (rose-coloured or white).

SWEETENERS
Small quantities of: honeydew honey, maple syrup*, dried fruit*, jaggery,* cane sugar*.

FRUIT
Pineapple, astringent apples, grapefruit, oranges, blueberries, pears, papaya, quince, rhubarb, dried fruit*, strawberries*, lemons*.

DRINKS
Teas: ginger, chai spices, green tea, fennel, rosehip, jasmine, chamomile, clove.

SUPPORTING **AGNI**

Good digestion is the key to our health. If you know and follow the rules of keeping your agni (digestive fire) strong, you will be happy and healthy, and enjoy the benefits of a good immune system.

Support your digestion

Agni is a fire that needs adequate fuel. Eating heavy foods and overeating are like putting wet wood or too much wood on the fire – it will be extinguished. If your agni is strong, you will feel light, nourished, and clear after a meal, and have no fatigue, heaviness, fullness, or indigestion.

Order, order

Heavy foods are harder to digest than light ones. Work with your digestion by eating different foods in the sequence below, which broadly corresponds with the order of the tastes (see p.62).

- **Heavy, oily, and hard** foods at the start.
- **Soft** foods next.
- **Light and liquid** foods at the end of the meal.

Yogurt, curd, and cheese

Yogurt and curd should not be eaten for dinner or at night as they will cause blockages. Hard cheeses are also heavy, oily, and cold and will have a similar effect.

The day and the seasons

Support your agni by tuning in to the natural rhythms of the day and the time of year, and working in harmony with them.

- **Agni is strongest** around noon and during winter; these are the times to eat heavier meals.
- **Agni is less active** in the morning and the evening, during summer, during illness, and immediately after exercise; these are the times to have light meals or fast (see p.86).

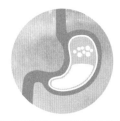

Improving digestion

The following practices will help create a strong agni.

- **Eat at** fixed times.
- **Eat only when** you are hungry.
- **Ensure meals are cooked** and eaten hot.
- **Make evening dinner** a light meal, and do not eat late.
- **Use plenty of spices.**
- **Consume** heavy, oily, fried, cold, and raw foods in small quantities only – they are hard to digest.
- **Fast one day** each week (see pp.86–87).
- **If you have fasted** for more than eight hours between meals, don't overload the stomach; this will put out your agni.
- **Do not drink cold water,** especially before, during, or after meals, and never add ice to your drinks.

> *"The period of life, complexion, strength, health, lustre, ojas, and energy are the result of the digestive fire."*
>
> SWAMI SIVANANDA

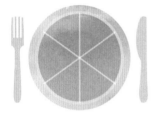

Mealtime guidelines

Your approach to mealtimes will affect your digestion. Take your time eating, chew well, and follow the order of the six tastes wherever possible (see p.62).

BEFORE MEALS

- **Be active** – take gentle exercise.
- **Eat 1–2 slices** of fresh ginger with lemon juice and rock salt, or chew a few fennel seeds.
- **Follow a ritual,** such as washing your hands and face and giving thanks (these can be unspoken).

AFTER MEALS

- **Chew a few** fennel seeds.
- **Take a walk** if possible.

Drinks for agni

To support agni, try the following drinks in the place of cold water.

AGNI DRINK

- **1 tsp** ground cumin
- **½ tsp** freshly ground black pepper (for pitta, you can use long pepper)
- **2–3 pinches** of ground ginger
- **pinch** of rock salt

Pour one cup of water into a saucepan. Add the spices and salt. Bring the seasoned water to the boil and simmer for 10 minutes. Pour into a cup and drink 30–45 minutes before your meal.

AYURVEDIC WATER

Boil water in an open saucepan for up to 20 minutes. Pour into a Thermos and drink throughout the day. Water boiled in this way is the most easily digestible form.

Agni and ojas

A strong agni will help to create ojas in the body (see pp.26–27). When agni is strong, the following foods increase ojas:

- **Milk** – drink 1 cup a day, warmed with spices and consumed hot
- **Ghee** – take up to 3 teaspoons a day
- **Almonds** – eat 3–4 a day, either roasted or soaked and peeled
- **Whole grains**
- **Ripe, sweet fruits.**

NOW MOVE TO
FASTING FOR HEALTH

FASTING FOR HEALTH

Fasting means giving up solid food in order to eliminate accumulated toxins and cleanse the system. It is a wonderful method of keeping healthy and activating self-healing.

Benefits of fasting

Fasting gives rest to the stomach, intestines and digestive organs. It cleanses and rejuvenates the body, removes blockages, relieves agni, and gives energy. Physically, your system gets an entire overhaul. Fasting will help you to develop strong willpower and enable you to concentrate better: it will also allow you to experience clarity.

How to fast

During a fast, drink plenty of hot water, herbal teas, or light broth. Don't do strenuous mental or physical work during any fast lasting 24 hours or longer. If you get nauseous, drink water mixed with a little lemon juice. Be careful not to give in to cravings or to overeat. If this happens, the best remedy is to fast again.

Breaking your fast

Break any fast that is longer than a day gradually, over the same duration as the fast. Reintroduce vegetable soup, diluted fruit juice, or coconut water first, three to four times daily for one-quarter of the length of the fast. Then, if your fast was longer than three days, continue with a diet of mainly fruit and cooked vegetables for the next few days.

16 HOURS

If your lifestyle or constitution doesn't allow for long fasts, this easy version is highly beneficial, especially when done on a regular basis.

Have a light lunch and then skip dinner or breakfast. This ensures a roughly 16-hour period of not eating solid foods.

A fast can vary in length from 16 hours to a few days. Seek the guidance of an expert if you wish to fast for longer than 2–3 days.

IMPORTANT NOTE

Talk to your doctor before fasting, especially if you have a health condition, or have had one in the past. Do not fast if you have an elevated vata, or you are pregnant, nursing, or underweight.

24 HOURS

During a 24-hour fast, drink hot water, hot agni drink (see p.85, use for increased kapha or if there is ama), or hot, light vegetable broth.

If it is too difficult to sustain the fast, you can mix the juice of 2–3 fruits with water, or drink 1–2 glasses of fresh carrot juice with a drop of vegetable oil.

Alternatively, try a 24-hour fruit fast. Any juicy fruit apart from mangoes will be beneficial. Avoid bananas and grapes.

2–3 DAYS

You can fast for as long as two or three days on your own, provided you are careful to break the fast slowly by gradually introducing light and soupy foods at the end of the fasting period.

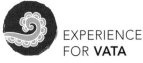

EXPERIENCE FOR **VATA**

People with elevated vata should not fast. Those with a lot of vata who are strong and healthy may start with a 16-hour fast.

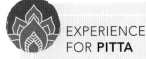

EXPERIENCE FOR **PITTA**

People with a lot of pitta benefit from fasting, as long as they are healthy, but may find it challenging to their active metabolism.

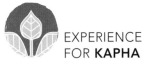

EXPERIENCE FOR **KAPHA**

Those with a lot of kapha in their constitution benefit most from fasting and should fast on a regular basis – ideally once a week.

COOKING AT HOME

The way you eat as well as what you eat can have a profound effect on your health. A positive, happy cook and a calm, relaxing environment are as important as the right foods.

Daily routine

Try to follow the guidance on this page and get into the habit of preparing regular, healthy meals suited to the season, your age, and – if required by an imbalance – your constitution.

- **Breakfast** should be nourishing, to give plenty of energy for the start of the day, but easy to digest: warm breakfasts are best.
- **Lunch** is the main meal and should be eaten between 11am and 2pm. If you don't have time to cook lunch, prepare it in the morning and bring it to work in a food flask.
- **Dinner** should be light, warm, and taken early evening. Avoid late, heavy meals.

Keep your food simple. Variation is good, but in moderation.

Your kitchen should be clean and the cook should be happy. **Stay positive, focused, and unhurried.**

Savour your food. *Chew slowly – digestion begins in the mouth.*

If you have an aversion to something it will have a negative effect on you, no matter how healthy you think it is. **Enjoy the food you eat.**

Take your time. *Eat sitting down.*

Eat in a peaceful atmosphere *without distractions, and focus on your food. Maintain silence if you can; otherwise keep the conversation light and positive.*

*When you
are stressed or
angry, calm yourself
with a few deep breaths
or wait a little
before eating.*

*Do not
eat or drink
anything that is
too hot or too cold.
Never use ice in
your drink.*

*Cook your own
food or have a loved one
cook for you if possible.
The mood of the cook
enters the food.*

*Buy fresh,
organic,
unprocessed
foods.*

*Eat moderately.
Overeating extinguishes
agni and produces ama. Eat
to live, don't live to eat,
and remember that food
is medicine.*

How to use the recipe pages

On the following pages you will find nutritious recipes for breakfasts, lunches, dinners, and desserts. These will help you gradually adapt your eating habits to be healthy and appropriate for your situation. If you wish to follow the order of the six tastes (see p.62), eat the grains first and the vegetables last. As salad is hard to digest and needs strong agni (digestive fire), it should also be eaten at the start of the meal. Some breakfast dishes may be suitable for lunch, or some lunches suitable for dinner; the key is to ensure you adapt portion sizes accordingly and keep breakfast and dinner light.

Adapting food by dosha

Many recipes offer a choice of ingredients. Use the dosha variation that is appropriate for the diet you are following. For more information about when to follow a diet for pacifying a specific dosha, see pp.72–73 (vata), pp.76–77 (pitta), or pp.80–81 (kapha). To determine if you have a dosha imbalance, see pp.48–49. If you are catering for several people, opt for a tridosha recipe, or one such as Vegetable Fritters (see p.109) where you can offer a selection of fritters to pacify different doshas.

Choosing ingredients

The ingredients should be available in your local supermarket or health food shop; source locally wherever possible. Milk is full fat, unless otherwise stated, and can be cows', goats', rice, or soy milk.

Equipment and storage

No special equipment is required to make the recipes, other than a food processor or hand-held blender for soups and chutneys. If you do not have a wok, use a heavy-based saucepan instead. Food should be eaten fresh, not stored or frozen.

Serves **5** | Prep time: **10 mins** | Cooking time: **30 mins**

SPICED RICE VERMICELLI

This spicy stir-fry makes a flavour-packed start to the day for any Ayurvedic diet. If you cannot get hold of curry leaves, use fresh coriander instead, as both pacify pitta and kapha.

INGREDIENTS

200g (7oz) rice vermicelli

4 tbsp vegetable oil or ghee

1 tsp black mustard seeds

2 tsp cumin seeds

2 tsp peeled and grated fresh root ginger

¼ tsp finely chopped green chilli; or pinch chilli powder

12 curry leaves (optional)

4 tbsp nuts or seeds by dosha
  - **VATA** cashew nuts
  - **PITTA** & **KAPHA** pumpkin seeds

4 tbsp desiccated coconut or shredded fresh coconut
  - **KAPHA** omit coconut

1 tsp ground turmeric

2 tsp salt, or to taste

200g (7oz) green peas or finely chopped green beans or mangetout

1 red pepper, deseeded and finely chopped

2 tbsp lemon juice

4 tbsp finely chopped coriander leaves, to garnish

1 Place the vermicelli in a heavy-based saucepan and pour in enough boiling water to cover completely. Cover with a lid and simmer for 3–5 minutes until the vermicelli is tender, then drain. If the noodles are very long, roughly chop or snip with scissors. Set aside to cool.

2 Heat the oil or ghee in a non-stick frying pan or large wok. When hot, add the mustard seeds and fry until they start to pop. Then add the cumin, ginger, chilli, curry leaves (if using), and cashew nuts or pumpkin seeds, and fry for 2–3 minutes until the nuts start to brown a little.

3 Add the coconut (if using) and stir. After 1 minute, add the turmeric, salt, and the vegetables. Pour in a little water, then cover and simmer for about 10 minutes on a medium heat until the vegetables are almost tender.

4 Add the cooked vermicelli to the vegetable mixture and stir-fry on a low heat for 3 minutes. Remove from the heat, sprinkle with the lemon juice, and transfer to a serving dish. Garnish with the coriander and serve hot.

Flavour

Frying spices in a little oil adds to their aroma and helps to unlock their active ingredients.

Serves **4** | Prep time: **5 mins** | Cooking time: **45 mins**

GRAIN PORRIDGE

The combination of milk and wholegrains in this dish makes it great for increasing ojas. It will also aid your digestion and keep you feeling satisfied for several hours, fending off any desire to snack before lunch.

INGREDIENTS

200g (7oz) grain by dosha, washed

- **VATA** amaranth or quinoa
- **PITTA** barley, amaranth, or quinoa
- **KAPHA** millet, barley, or quinoa

4 tbsp raisins

4 tbsp sunflower seeds

1 tsp ground cardamom

4 tbsp sweetener by dosha, to taste

- **VATA & PITTA** demerara sugar, or agave or rice syrup
- **KAPHA** raw honey or concentrated apple juice

400ml (14fl oz) milk by dosha

- **VATA & PITTA** full-fat milk
- **KAPHA** skimmed milk

1 Place the grain of your choice into a heavy-based saucepan. Add 800ml (1½ pints) cold water (400ml/14fl oz water if using amaranth) and bring to the boil. Reduce the heat and simmer for 15 minutes if using amaranth, 25 minutes if using quinoa, and 45 minutes if using barley or millet, stirring occasionally in each case and adding more water to the barley if necessary.

2 Add the raisins, seeds, and cardamom, and cook for another 2 minutes.

3 Divide the porridge between 4 bowls, add your sweetener of choice, and finally add 100ml (3½fl oz) milk to each bowl.

Honey

If you are using honey, add it once the porridge has cooled down a little. According to Ayurveda, honey causes ama (toxins) if heated above 40°C (104°F).

WHOLEGRAIN PANCAKES

These fluffy, wholegrain pancakes are filling and easy to make. Baking powder with sparkling water and milk are used as the raising agent so that this breakfast is suitable for a sattvic diet.

INGREDIENTS

360g (12½oz) flour by dosha
- **VATA** & **PITTA** spelt or wholewheat flour
- **KAPHA 270g (9½oz)** buckwheat flour, plus **90g (3oz)** rice flour

4 tsp baking powder

pinch salt, or to taste

300ml (10fl oz) milk, or enough to make a thick batter

300ml (10fl oz) sparkling water, or enough to make a thick batter

4 tbsp ghee, melted, or vegetable oil

FOR THE TOPPINGS

Toppings by dosha, to taste
- **VATA** maple or agave syrup, toasted cashews or blanched almonds
- **PITTA** maple or agave syrup, toasted sunflower or pumpkin seeds
- **KAPHA** raw honey or apple juice, toasted sunflower or pumpkin seeds

1 Preheat the oven to 130°C (250°F/Gas ½). Mix your flour of choice with the baking powder and salt. Gradually add just enough milk and sparkling water to make a thick batter. You may need all the liquid for the kapha variation, but only about 300ml (10fl oz) for the vata and pitta variations. Combine very lightly with a whisk to ensure the pancakes remain fluffy. Don't worry if the batter is still a little lumpy.

2 Heat some of the ghee or oil in a non-stick frying pan. Test the temperature by adding a spoonful of batter to the pan. It should sizzle without burning, and after 1–2 minutes bubbles should form.

3 Pour a small ladleful of batter into the pan to make an American-style pancake if you are cooking for vata or pitta, or a thin, crêpe-style pancake if you are kapha. Drizzle a little ghee or oil around the edges, and cook until bubbles form on the surface, or until the edges stiffen (about 2 minutes). Then flip the pancake, drizzle with more ghee or oil, and cook for another 90 seconds.

4 Keep the finished pancakes on a baking sheet in the warm oven while you cook the rest. Add more ghee or oil to the pan as required. Serve with the toppings.

Thickness

Vata is pacified by thick pancakes and pitta by medium-thickness pancakes. To pacify kapha, eat a half portion or make crêpe-style versions by spreading the batter thinly when cooking.

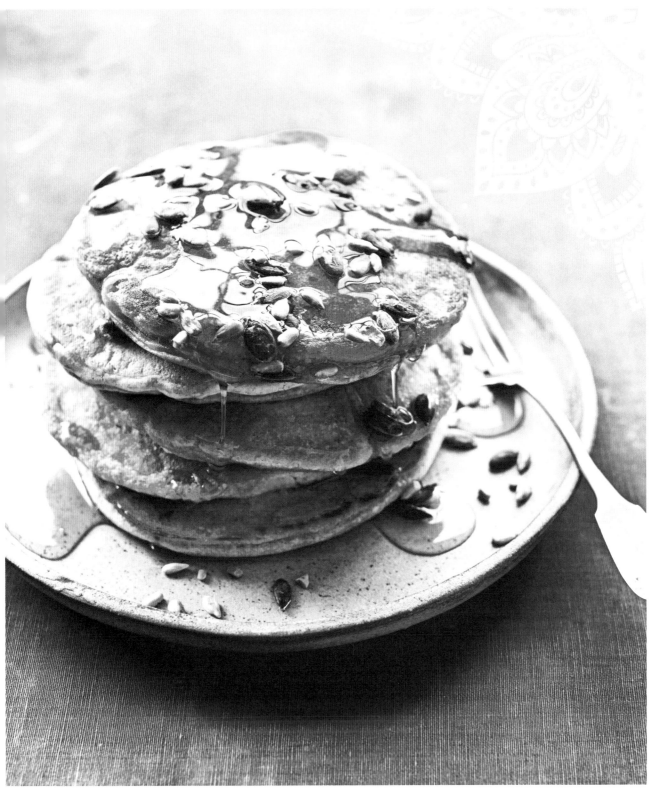

▲ Pitta variation

BREAKFAST SPREADS

Eat these spreads on wholegrain toast as an easy way to adapt your breakfast to a diet that pacifies a specific dosha – simply choose the spread most relevant to you.

Serves **4** | Prep time: **15** mins

VATA SPREAD

INGREDIENTS

3 beetroots, peeled and finely grated

1 large avocado, mashed

4 tsp ghee, or olive or sesame oil

2 tbsp cashews, finely chopped

3 tbsp lemon juice, or to taste

4 tbsp chopped basil

1 tsp salt, or to taste

pinch of freshly ground black pepper

The sweet vegetables and ghee in this spread pacify vata. Those eating for vata benefit from warm foods, so eat on warm toast or pancakes with a cup of hot, herbal tea.

1 Gently combine all the ingredients in a mixing bowl, or use a food processor to blend them until you have a spreadable paste.

Serves **4** | Prep time: **15** mins

PITTA SPREAD

INGREDIENTS

1 cucumber, peeled, deseeded, finely grated, and the water squeezed out

35g (1¼oz) rocket, finely chopped

1 large avocado, mashed

4 tsp ghee or coconut oil

2 tbsp sunflower seeds, crushed, or fresh coconut, shredded

3 tbsp lemon juice, or to taste

2 tbsp chopped mint (optional)

1 tsp salt, or to taste

Cucumbers and coconut are cooling, while rocket is bitter and cooling, so all three pacify pitta. Allow the toast to cool before eating.

1 Gently combine all the ingredients in a mixing bowl, or use a food processor to blend them until you have a spreadable paste.

Serves **4** | Prep time: **15** mins

KAPHA SPREAD

The bitter salad greens and a touch of hot spice in this spread pacify kapha. Choose yeast-free bread and eat on warm toast.

INGREDIENTS

70g (2½oz) rocket, finely chopped

2 sticks celery, finely chopped

1 large avocado, mashed

2 tsp ghee or linseed oil

2 tbsp pumpkin seeds, crushed

½ tsp freshly ground black pepper

pinch of chilli powder

3 tbsp lemon juice, or to taste

1 tsp salt, or to taste

1 Gently combine all the ingredients in a mixing bowl, or use a food processor to blend them until you have a spreadable paste.

Serves **4** | Prep time: **5 mins**, plus soaking

TRIDOSHA SPREAD

This uncooked prune spread is a healthy way to satisfy a sweet tooth. It is good for all three doshas, but kapha should take care to consume in moderation.

INGREDIENTS

100g (3½oz) prunes, rinsed and pitted

4 dried figs, rinsed and trimmed at the ends

8 dates, rinsed and pitted

1 tsp ground cinnamon

1 Place the dried fruits in a bowl with 300ml (10fl oz) water. Leave to soak overnight.

2 Strain the dried fruits. Place in a food processor with the cinnamon and half the soaking water, then blend to a smooth paste. Alternatively, use a hand-held blender. This spread will keep for up to one week in the fridge.

LUNCHES

Serves **6–8** | Prep time: **20 mins** | Cooking time: **45–60 mins**

MEDITERRANEAN VEGETABLE GRATIN *with crisp salad*

This gratin nourishes those with a lot of vata in their constitution. Those with a lot of pitta benefit from its combination with the raw salad, while those with a lot of kapha can indulge if they reduce the amount of cheese.

INGREDIENTS

4 firm, ripe tomatoes

2 tbsp olive oil

12 medium potatoes, peeled and sliced

4 carrots, peeled and cut into sticks

4 fennel bulbs, thickly sliced

1 bunch Swiss chard, chopped

500g (1lb 2oz) ricotta cheese
   • **KAPHA** 200g (7oz)

250ml (9fl oz) milk

3 tsp salt, or to taste

¾ tsp freshly ground black pepper

1½ tsp ground nutmeg

3 tbsp finely chopped fresh rosemary leaves

3 tbsp finely chopped fresh sage leaves

300g (10oz) mozzarella cheese, thinly sliced

4 tsp pine nuts

8 black olives, pitted, to garnish

½ bunch basil, to garnish

MAIN DISH

VEGETABLE GRATIN

1 Preheat the oven to 200ºC (400ºF/Gas 6). Soak the tomatoes in a bowl of boiling water for 2 minutes, then remove their skins. Slice thinly.

2 Grease a large roasting tin with the oil. Arrange the sliced potatoes in a layer at the bottom of the tin. Add the carrot sticks to form the next layer, then the fennel, and then the Swiss chard. Set the tin aside.

3 Whisk the ricotta cheese and milk into a creamy sauce and add the salt and pepper, nutmeg, rosemary, and sage. Pour the sauce into the roasting tin over the vegetable and potato layers. Layer the sauce with the sliced tomatoes and mozzarella.

4 Cover with foil and bake for 45–60 minutes, or until cooked through. Ten minutes before the end, remove the foil and sprinkle the pine nuts over the gratin. When the nuts and cheese have browned, remove the gratin from the oven and garnish with the black olives and basil leaves.

Adding salad

Salad and raw foods are particularly beneficial to pitta in the summertime. If you are eating for elevated vata or kapha, it is advisable to keep portions modest or avoid salad.

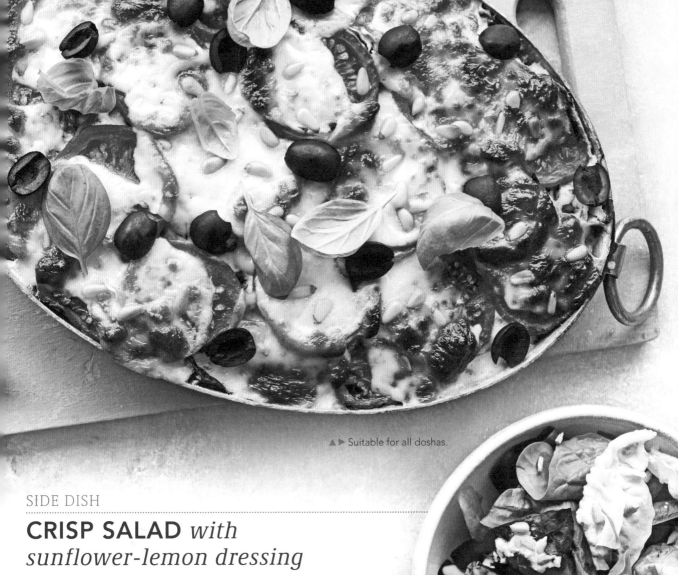

▲ ▶ Suitable for all doshas.

SIDE DISH

CRISP SALAD *with* *sunflower-lemon dressing*

INGREDIENTS

4 tbsp sunflower seeds

4 tbsp lemon juice

½ tsp salt, or to taste

pinch of freshly ground black pepper

1 bowlful assorted salad leaves, washed

1 Blend the sunflower seeds, lemon juice, salt, pepper, and 60ml (2fl oz) water to a smooth consistency, adding more water if necessary. Set aside.

2 Place the salad in a bowl and drizzle over the dressing.

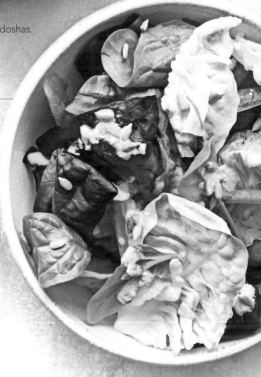

LUNCHES

Serves **4** | Prep time: **15 mins** | Cooking time: **40 mins**

BAKED CUMIN POTATOES
with courgettes and hummus

This nourishing dish is served with hummus, an alternative, dosha-adaptable way of adding pulses to your diet. Hummus also serves as a light meal when eaten with wholegrain toast.

INGREDIENTS

4 tbsp vegetable oil

2 tsp salt, or to taste

pinch of chilli powder

4 medium courgettes, washed, trimmed, and halved lengthways

2 tsp fennel seeds, crushed

2 tsp ground cumin

12 medium potatoes, well scrubbed and halved lengthways

MAIN DISH

BAKED CUMIN POTATOES
with courgettes

1 Preheat the oven to 200°C (400°F/Gas 6). Mix the oil with the salt and chilli, then rub half the mixture onto the courgettes. Sprinkle the courgettes with the crushed fennel seeds.

2 Stir the ground cumin into the remaining oil mixture and rub the mixture onto the potatoes.

3 Arrange the potatoes and the courgettes on two separate baking trays. Place the potatoes in the oven to bake. After about 10 minutes, put the courgettes in the oven. Bake for 30 minutes, or until both the potatoes and courgettes are tender. Serve with hummus.

Dip it

You could try cutting the potatoes and courgettes into chip shapes before baking, and then dipping them into the hummus when cooked.

SIDE DISH

HUMMUS

INGREDIENTS

160g (5¾oz) legumes by dosha, well rinsed

- **VATA** yellow mung dhal
- **PITTA & KAPHA** dried chickpeas, soaked overnight

3 tbsp nut paste by dosha

- **VATA** tahini
- **PITTA** almond butter, or double olive oil
- **KAPHA** 2 tbsp tahini

4 tbsp olive oil

- **KAPHA** 2 tbsp

pinch of chilli powder

- **KAPHA** 2 pinches

1 tsp salt, or to taste

4 tbsp lemon juice, or to taste

1 tsp paprika

4 tbsp chopped basil or coriander, to garnish

8 black olives, pitted, to garnish

1 Place the mung dhal or chickpeas in a saucepan of water. Use plenty of water for the chickpeas and just enough to sit 2cm above the surface of the mung dhal. Bring to the boil. Reduce the heat and simmer until soft (about 30 minutes for the mung dhal, and about 90 minutes for the chickpeas). If using mung dhal, add more hot water during cooking if necessary. Strain, retaining some of the cooking water.

2 Blend the legumes, nut paste, oil, chilli, salt, lemon juice, and reserved cooking water into a creamy paste.

3 Transfer the hummus into a bowl, sprinkle with the paprika, and garnish with the herbs and black olives.

Mung dhal

If cooking for vata, don't use a blender, as the mung dhal will break up as it cooks. Whisk all the ingredients together, adding a little water if necessary.

LUNCHES

Serves **4** | Prep time: **15 mins** | Cooking time: **25 mins**

KHICHDI *with raita*

This rice-and-lentil dish, accompanied by a refreshing raita, is a classic meal for a sattvic diet. Make the raita first (or in advance) and set aside. The khichdi will swell up during cooking, so make sure you use a large enough pan.

INGREDIENTS

160g (5¾oz) rice by dosha, well rinsed

- **VATA** white basmati rice
- **PITTA** brown basmati rice
- **KAPHA** brown rice, soaked overnight

80g (2¾oz) yellow mung dhal, well rinsed

2 tsp ground turmeric

8 green cardamom pods

½ tsp black peppercorns

1 cinnamon stick (or **½ tsp** ground cinnamon)

400g (14oz) vegetables by dosha, washed and diced

- **VATA** equal parts peeled carrots, courgettes, and fennel
- **PITTA** equal parts cauliflower, spinach, and sweet potatoes
- **KAPHA** equal parts broccoli, carrots, and Swiss chard

2 tsp salt, or to taste

2 tbsp olive oil or ghee

2 tsp cumin seeds

4 tsp peeled and grated fresh root ginger

2 tsp curry powder (garlic-free)

2 tbsp lemon juice

2 tbsp coriander leaves, to garnish

MAIN DISH

KHICHDI

1 Put the rice and mung dhal into a large, heavy-based saucepan. Add the turmeric, cardamom, peppercorns, cinnamon, and 900ml (1½ pints) cold water. Cover and bring to the boil, then reduce the heat and simmer for 10 minutes.

2 Add the diced vegetables and the salt, cover again, and simmer for another 10 minutes until soft. If you are using spinach or broccoli and Swiss chard, leave these out and add them during the final 2–5 minutes of cooking.

3 Heat the oil or ghee in a small saucepan and fry the cumin seeds until they are golden brown. Then add the ginger and, after a few seconds, the curry powder. Remove from the heat and gently stir the spices into the rice and mung dhal mixture.

4 Sprinkle with the lemon juice, garnish with the coriander, and serve accompanied by raita.

▶ Pitta-kapha variation

Texture

Traditionally, khichdi is a creamy dish which is suited to all constitutions. Here we show a pitta-kapha variation with lots of vegetables for kapha and fimly cooked rice and dhal for Pitta's strong digestive fire.

SIDE DISH
RAITA

INGREDIENTS

2 tsp cumin seeds

1 cucumber, about 200g (7oz), peeled and grated

250g (9oz) yogurt by dosha
- **VATA** & **PITTA** full-fat
- **KAPHA** low-fat

1 tsp salt, or to taste

4 tbsp finely chopped coriander leaves

1 Toast the cumin seeds in a pan on a medium heat until they become fragrant and turn a shade darker. Grind to a powder using a mortar and pestle or an electric coffee mill.

2 Combine the grated cucumber, yogurt, salt, and ground cumin in a bowl. Sprinkle with coriander.

▶ Raita is suitable for all doshas, especially pitta

Cucumber

Grate the cucumber onto kitchen paper. This will soak up any excess water that could make the raita too loose.

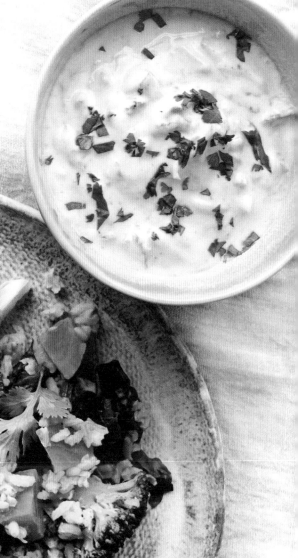

Serves **4** | Prep time: **10 mins** | Cooking time: **45–90 mins**

SIMPLE DHAL *with grains and almond vegetables*

Grains, vegetables, pulses, and fats are the four core foods that the body requires. A simple dhal served with grains and vegetables is the most popular form of lunch in ayurvedic cuisine as it contains all of these foods.

INGREDIENTS

160g (5¾oz) pulses by dosha, well rinsed

- **VATA** yellow mung dhal, split green mung dhal, or red lentils
- **PITTA** chana dhal, whole green mung dhal, or dried green lentils, soaked overnight and drained
- **KAPHA** dried chickpeas, toor dhal, or aduki beans, soaked overnight and drained

1 tsp ground turmeric

200g (7oz) spinach or the green part of Swiss chard, washed and torn

1 tsp salt, or to taste

3 tsp lemon juice

4 tsp finely chopped coriander leaves

FOR THE GRAINS
200g (7oz) grains by dosha

- **VATA** bulgur wheat, quinoa, or white Basmati rice
- **PITTA** barley, brown Basmati rice, or bulgur wheat
- **KAPHA** barley, brown rice, or buckwheat

½ tsp salt

FOR THE CURRY PASTE
4 tsp vegetable oil or ghee

1 tsp cumin seeds

3 tsp peeled and finely chopped fresh root ginger

⅛ green chilli, or pinch of chilli powder

1 tsp ground cumin

1 tsp ground coriander

2 tsp curry powder (garlic-free) or garam masala

1 tsp turmeric

MAIN DISH

SIMPLE DHAL *with grains*

1 Place the legumes into a large saucepan with 700ml (1¼ pints) water and the turmeric, then bring to the boil. Remove any foam with a slotted spoon, reduce the heat, and cover. Vata legumes take about 30 minutes, pitta about 60 minutes, and kapha about 75 minutes. Add more hot water if needed. When the legumes are soft, add the leafy vegetables and salt. Simmer for a further 10 minutes, then remove the pan from the heat.

2 Add the grain to a medium saucepan with 460ml (15½ fl oz) water (700ml/1¼ pints for brown rice) and the salt, cover, then bring to the boil. Reduce the heat and simmer until done – do not stir or uncover. White Basmati, quinoa, and bulgur wheat take about 20 minutes; brown Basmati and barley about 30 minutes; and brown rice and buckwheat about 60 minutes. Drain.

3 For the curry paste, heat the oil or ghee in a small frying pan, then add the cumin seeds, ginger, and chilli. After a few seconds, add the ground cumin, coriander, curry powder, and turmeric and heat briefly. As soon as the spices are fragrant, remove the pan from the heat and stir in 3 tablespoons of water. The hot pan will make the water evaporate, leaving a paste.

4 Stir the curry paste into the cooked legumes, then add the lemon juice and garnish with the coriander. Serve the dhal with the grain and almond vegetables.

SIDE DISH

ALMOND VEGETABLES

INGREDIENTS

800g (1¾lb) vegetables by dosha, washed, peeled, and diced

- **VATA** beetroots, parsnips, and sweet potatoes
- **PITTA** broccoli, carrots, and green beans
- **KAPHA** cabbage, cauliflower, and green beans

2 tsp ground turmeric

8 tbsp ground almonds

4 tbsp vegetable oil

2 tsp ground cumin

8 curry leaves (optional)

1 tsp salt, or to taste

½ tsp freshly ground black pepper

2 tsp lemon juice

1 Place the vegetables in a saucepan with 250ml (9fl oz) water and the turmeric. Bring to the boil, then reduce the heat and simmer for about 10 minutes until tender.

2 Stir in the ground almonds, oil, cumin, curry leaves (if using), and salt and pepper, and cook for another 2 minutes, adding more hot water if necessary. Remove from the heat and sprinkle with the lemon juice.

Purifying

Vegetables that are low in starch are purifying foods, which means that they help reduce any excess tissue and pacify kapha.

STIR-FRIED VEGETABLES
with sesame noodles

Take care not to overcook this crisp stir-fry. Tender vegetables benefit those with dominant vata or kapha, while those with dominant pitta will benefit from (and may enjoy) eating them *al dente*.

INGREDIENTS

250g (9oz) firm tofu, cut into cubes

6 tbsp soy sauce, to taste

2 tsp ground cumin

2 pinches of chilli powder

1 tsp ground ginger

6 tbsp vegetable oil

4 tbsp peeled and grated fresh root ginger

½ tsp freshly ground black pepper

1 tsp ground nutmeg

1 tsp ground cinnamon

800g (1¾lb) vegetables by dosha, washed and thinly sliced

- **VATA** equal parts courgettes, Swiss chard, and carrots

- **PITTA** equal parts white cabbage, spinach, and red peppers

- **KAPHA** equal parts pak choi (quartered, not sliced), beansprouts (whole), and red peppers

1 stalk of lemongrass, cut in half length-wise, or 2 tsp lemon zest

4 tsp sesame oil (optional)

4 tbsp basil, shredded, to serve

MAIN DISH

STIR-FRIED VEGETABLES

1 Marinate the tofu for at least 10 minutes in 2 tablespoons of soy sauce, 1 teaspoon of cumin, a pinch of chilli powder, and the ground ginger.

2 Heat 4 tablespoons of oil in a wok. Add 2 tablespoons of grated ginger and fry for 30 seconds. Then add the black pepper, nutmeg, cinnamon, and the remaining cumin and chilli powder. Immediately, add the sliced vegetables, with the exception of the beansprouts (if using), together with the remaining soy sauce, a little water, and the stalk of lemongrass (if using).

3 Stir-fry the vegetables until they are cooked according to dosha: vata, well cooked; pitta, slightly undercooked; and kapha, just crisp or *al dente* (about 12 minutes). If using beansprouts, add these in the final 2 minutes of cooking. Remove from the heat and add the remaining grated ginger. If you are using grated lemon zest, add it now.

4 Heat the remaining oil in a non-stick pan and fry the tofu with the marinade over a medium heat until it turns golden brown and crisp. Add this to the vegetables.

5 Add more soy sauce to taste if required, sprinkle with roasted sesame oil (if using, avoid adding oil here if cooking for those with dominant kapha), and add the basil to serve.

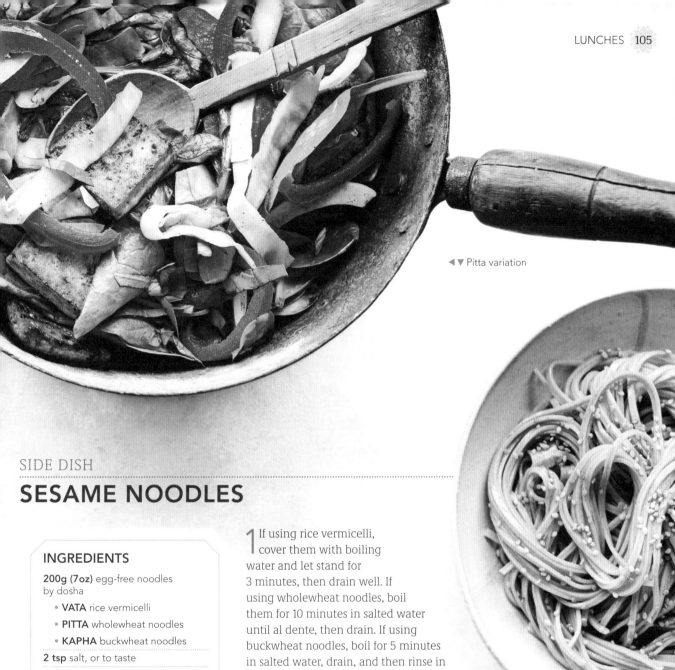

◄▼ Pitta variation

SIDE DISH

SESAME NOODLES

INGREDIENTS

200g (7oz) egg-free noodles
by dosha

- **VATA** rice vermicelli
- **PITTA** wholewheat noodles
- **KAPHA** buckwheat noodles

2 tsp salt, or to taste

4 tbsp brown sesame seeds

2 tbsp vegetable oil (optional)

1 If using rice vermicelli, cover them with boiling water and let stand for 3 minutes, then drain well. If using wholewheat noodles, boil them for 10 minutes in salted water until al dente, then drain. If using buckwheat noodles, boil for 5 minutes in salted water, drain, and then rinse in cold water. Drizzle with oil (if using).

2 Toast the sesame seeds in a frying pan over a medium heat until they become fragrant and turn a shade darker. Sprinkle over the noodles, mix well, and serve.

DINNERS

ALOO METHI
with mango chutney

This potato dish with fenugreek leaves makes a light dinner suitable for all doshas, or can be used to accompany a lunch of curry or dhal. It contains five of the six tastes (only astringent is missing), making it a well-rounded Ayurvedic meal.

INGREDIENTS

4 tbsp ghee or vegetable oil

12 medium potatoes, peeled and diced

2 tsp ground turmeric

2 tsp salt, or to taste

pinch of chilli powder

8 tbsp dried fenugreek leaves (kasoori methi), soaked in water for 5 minutes, or finely chopped coriander leaves

4 tbsp lemon juice

For the chutney

1 ripe mango, peeled, stoned, and cut into cubes

pinch of chilli powder

½ tsp salt, or to taste

4 tsp lemon juice

2 tsp agave syrup

2 tsp ghee or vegetable oil

1 tsp black mustard seeds

1 Start by making the chutney. Purée the mango, chilli powder, salt, lemon juice, and agave syrup with a little water using a food processor or hand-held blender.

2 Heat the ghee or oil in a small frying pan over a medium heat. Add the mustard seeds and fry until they start to pop. Remove from the heat, add to the mango purée, and set aside.

3 Next make the aloo methi. In a heavy-based saucepan, heat the ghee or oil. When hot, add the potatoes, along with the turmeric, salt, and chilli powder, and sauté for a few minutes.

4 Add the fenugreek leaves (if using) and some of the soaking water. Cover and simmer over a low heat for 20 minutes, or until the potatoes are cooked through. If you are using fresh coriander, add it at the end of the cooking time.

5 Remove from the heat, sprinkle with the lemon juice, and transfer to a serving dish. Serve hot, with a dollop of the mango chutney. The chutney will keep for 3 days in the fridge.

Serves **4** | Prep time: **10 mins** | Cooking time: **15 mins**

CREAMY SQUASH SOUP

Quick to make and delicious to eat, this soup makes the perfect light, easily digestible, tridosha meal for a 6pm dinner. This means it will be fully digested by the time you go to bed, and won't affect your sleep.

INGREDIENTS

4 tbsp ghee
- **KAPHA** olive or rapeseed oil

1 large butternut squash, peeled, deseeded, and diced

4 medium potatoes, peeled and cut into cubes

1 tsp grated nutmeg

2 tsp salt, or to taste

½ tsp freshly ground black pepper

4 tbsp finely chopped dill

2 tbsp lemon juice

1 Heat the ghee or oil in a large saucepan. Add the squash and potatoes, and stir-fry for a few minutes.

2 Cover with cold water, then add the nutmeg and salt and pepper, and bring to the boil. Cover and simmer for 10–15 minutes on a low heat until the vegetables are tender.

3 Using a food processor or hand-held blender, purée most of the vegetables to make a creamy soup, leaving a few chunks. Stir in the dill and lemon juice before serving.

Colour

Stir in the dill, rather than blend it, in order not to dull the vibrant colour of the soup.

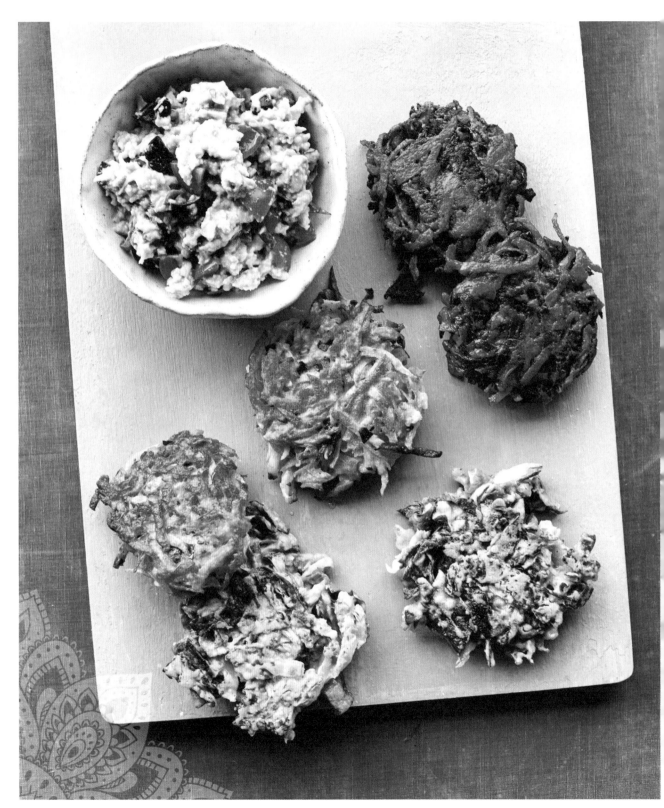

▲ Pitta (middle), kapha (bottom), and vata (top right) variations with avocado dip (top)

Makes **10** fritters | Prep time: **10 mins** | Cooking time: **15–20 mins**

VEGETABLE FRITTERS
with avocado-olive dip

These crispy fritters make for a colourful dinner table if you are catering for several different doshas. Make a batch of each type so that there is an option for everyone, and serve with the avocado dip.

INGREDIENTS

900g (2lb) vegetables by dosha, peeled and grated, shredded, or finely diced

• **VATA** equal parts beetroots and sweet potatoes

• **PITTA** equal parts celeriac and carrots

• **KAPHA** equal parts cabbage and spinach

45g (1½oz) chickpea flour, sifted

2 tsp salt, or to taste

½ tsp freshly ground black pepper

½ tsp grated nutmeg

bunch fresh parsley, finely chopped

4 tbsp vegetable oil

FOR THE DIP

2 ripe, medium avocados

3 tbsp lemon juice, plus 1 slice of lemon to garnish

4 cherry tomatoes, diced

4 tbsp finely chopped basil, plus leaves to garnish

10 black olives, pitted and quartered, plus extra to garnish

4 tsp olive oil

½ tsp salt, or to taste

pinch freshly ground black pepper

1 Start by making the dip. Halve and stone the avocados, scoop out the pulp with a spoon, then mash with a fork. Immediately sprinkle over the lemon juice.

2 Gently fold in the tomatoes, basil, olives, oil, and salt and pepper. Garnish with a lemon slice, a few olives, and basil leaves. Set aside.

3 To make the fritters, combine the vegetables, flour, salt and pepper, nutmeg, and parsley with enough water for the mixture to hold when you press it together. If it doesn't hold, add more flour. Don't let the mixture sit for a long time as it will become too runny.

4 Preheat the oven to 130°C (250°F/Gas ½). Heat the oil in a non-stick frying pan. Shape the mixture into 10 patties and place several into the pan. Fry the fritters slowly over a medium heat for about 4 minutes on each side. Adjust the heat so that the fritters gently sizzle and the insides cook without the outsides burning. Briefly drain the fritters on kitchen paper, then place them on a baking sheet in the warm oven while you use up the remaining mixture. Serve warm with the avocado dip.

Low fat

Alternatively, you can place the fritters on a greased baking tray, drizzle them with the remaining oil, and bake them in the oven for 25–30 minutes at 200°C (100°F/Gas 6).

DINNERS

RICE PULAO
with ginger-raisin chutney

Rice cooked with vegetables and spices is easy to prepare after a long day at work. Adding a small amount of chutney to your plate is a good way to get more of the six tastes into your meal: this chutney is sweet, sour, and pungent.

INGREDIENTS

4 tbsp ghee or vegetable oil

200g (7oz) white or brown Basmati rice, soaked in water for 30 minutes; then drained

400g (14oz) vegetables by dosha, finely diced

- **VATA** equal parts green peas (whole) and carrots
- **PITTA** equal parts cauliflower and green peppers
- **KAPHA** equal parts green beans and red peppers

4 tbsp nuts or seeds by dosha

- **VATA** cashews or blanched almonds
- **PITTA** blanched almonds
- **KAPHA** pumpkin seeds

4 tbsp raisins or chopped dates (optional)

2 tsp salt, or to taste

8 black peppercorns

2 tsp ground turmeric

1 cinnamon stick

8 green cardamom pods

4 bay leaves

4 tbsp coarsely chopped coriander leaves

4 tbsp lemon juice

lemon wedges, to garnish

FOR THE CHUTNEY

8 tbsp raisins

4 tbsp peeled and finely chopped fresh root ginger

pinch of chilli powder

- **KAPHA** 2 pinches

2 tbsp lemon juice, or to taste

sprig of coriander, to garnish

1 lemon wedge, to garnish

1 Heat the ghee or oil in a heavy-based saucepan. Add the rice and stir-fry for 2 minutes.

2 Add the vegetables, nuts or seeds, raisins or dates (if using), salt, peppercorns, turmeric, cinnamon, cardamom pods, and bay leaves and stir-fry for a further 3 minutes.

3 Add 260ml (9fl oz) cold water, bring to the boil, cover, and simmer on a low heat. Do not stir or lift the lid until the rice is cooked and has absorbed the water (about 15 minutes for white Basmati and 25 minutes for brown Basmati).

4 Make the chutney. Blend the raisins, ginger, chilli powder, and lemon juice in a small food processor to a creamy paste, or mash with a fork if necessary. Garnish with the coriander and lemon wedge and set aside.

5 Sprinkle the coriander and lemon juice over the pulao and garnish with lemon wedges. Serve with the chutney.

Chutneys

These are side dishes that spruce up a simple meal and support digestion. They should only be eaten in small quantities.

Serves **4** | Prep time: **20 mins** | Cooking time: **25 mins**

MIXED VEGETABLE SOUP

This soup is an ideal meal if your agni needs strengthening. It is light and packed full of spices, and the vegetables are well cooked. Eating before 6pm will ensure that you can digest your food properly before going to bed.

INGREDIENTS

4 tbsp vegetable oil or ghee by dosha

- **VATA & PITTA** vegetable oil or ghee
- **KAPHA** vegetable oil

600g (1lb 5oz) vegetables by dosha, peeled and diced, or shredded

- **VATA** equal parts fennel, sweet potatoes, and mangetout
- **PITTA** equal parts broccoli, carrots, and celeriac
- **VATA** equal parts kale, parsnips, and red peppers

2 tsp salt, or to taste

4 bay leaves

2 tsp ground turmeric

2 tsp ground cumin

1 tsp ground coriander

1 tsp ground ginger

pinch of chilli powder

pinch of ground cloves

½ tsp ground cinnamon

4 tsp lemon juice

4 tbsp shredded coriander leaves or parsley

1 Heat the oil or ghee in a large saucepan. Add the vegetables (apart from the mangetout, broccoli or kale if using), salt, bay leaves, and all the spices, and stir-fry for a few minutes.

2 Add 800ml (1½ pints) cold water to the pan. Bring to the boil, cover, and simmer on a low heat for 10–15 minutes, or until the vegetables are tender. Add the green vegetables 5 minutes before the end.

3 Remove from the heat, discard the bay leaves, and add the lemon juice and coriander or parsley. Serve with toast or boiled grains.

Spices

For best results, measure out the spices before you start cooking, so that you can add them to the pan simultaneously.

DINNERS

Serves **4** | Prep time: **10 mins** | Cooking time: **15 mins**

WHOLEGRAIN PASTA
with pesto sauce

Here, a Western favourite is adapted by dosha, proving how easy eating a specific dosha diet can be. It contains all six tastes – the pasta is sweet, the cheese sour and salty, and the herbs pungent, bitter, and astringent.

INGREDIENTS

400g (14oz) egg-free pasta by dosha

- **VATA** spelt pasta
- **PITTA** wholewheat pasta
- **KAPHA** buckwheat noodles

1 tsp salt

FOR THE PESTO SAUCE

4 tbsp nuts or seeds by dosha

- **VATA** equal parts pine nuts and cashews
- **PITTA** equal parts blanched almonds and pumpkin seeds
- **KAPHA** equal parts sunflower seeds and pumpkin seeds

4 tbsp ricotta cheese

4 tbsp olive oil

bunch basil, coarsely chopped

4 tbsp sage leaves

4 tbsp rosemary leaves

2 tsp salt, or to taste

½ tsp freshly ground black pepper

4 tsp lemon juice

200g (7oz) Parmesan cheese, grated (optional)

1 Boil the pasta in a large saucepan of salted water, according to the instructions on the packet, until al dente. Strain and set aside.

2 To make the pesto, toast the nuts or seeds in a frying pan until fragrant.

3 Blend the toasted nuts or seeds, ricotta, oil, herbs, salt and pepper, lemon juice, and a little cooking water into a smooth, creamy paste using a food processor or hand-held blender.

4 Mix the pasta with the pesto sauce and a little cooking water. Sprinkle with the Parmesan (if using) and serve.

Fresh herbs

The fresher the basil, sage, and rosemary, the better, as fresher foods provide more sattva.

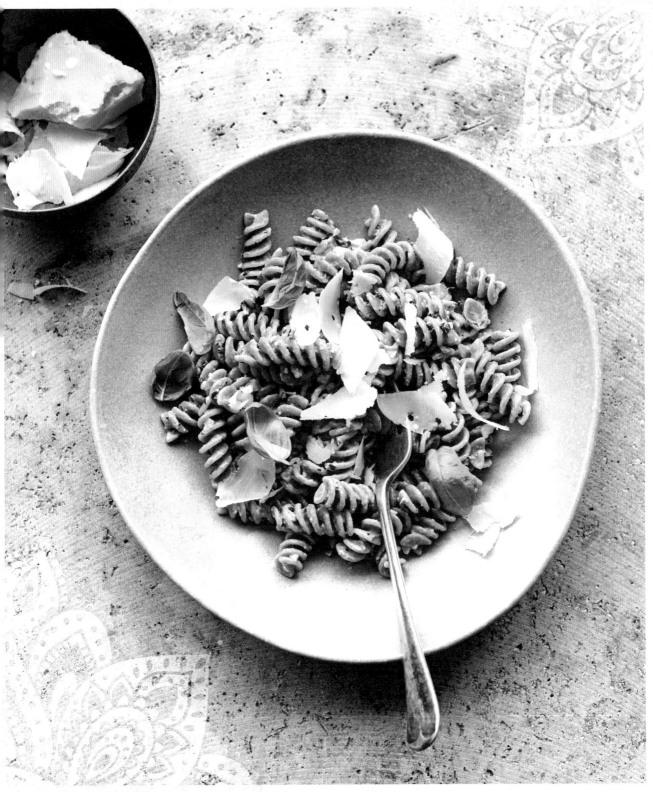

▲ Vata variation

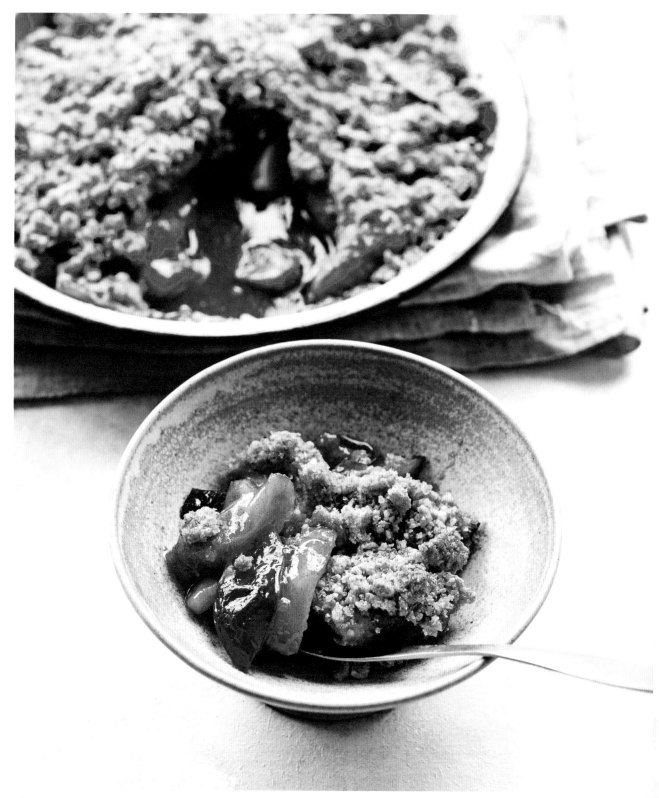

▲ Pitta variation

DESSERTS   Serves **6** | Prep time: **15 mins** | Cooking time: **40 mins**

FRUIT CRUMBLE

Fruit should be cooked when it is being eaten as part of a meal because
this makes it more easily digestible. Crumble is a delicious way to include
a variety of fruits in your diet.

INGREDIENTS

FOR THE FILLING

450g (1lb) fresh fruits by dosha,
cleaned, peeled, and stoned, or
cored and diced

- **VATA** equal parts sweet
  apples and peaches or plums
- **PITTA** equal parts sweet
  apples and sweet plums
- **KAPHA** equal parts pears
  and apricots

40g (1¼oz) demerara sugar

1 tbsp cornflour

1 tbsp ground cinnamon

1 pinch of freshly ground
black pepper

2 tbsp lemon juice

FOR THE CRUMBLE

200g (7oz) butter or margarine,
cut into cubes, plus extra
for greasing

300g (10oz) wholegrain flour

- **VATA** spelt flour
- **PITTA** wholewheat flour
- **KAPHA** buckwheat flour

175g (6oz) demerara sugar

2 tsp vanilla essence

pinch of salt

1 Preheat the oven to 180°C (350°F/Gas 4). Grease
a baking dish with some butter or margarine.

2 To make the filling, gently mix together the fruit,
sugar, cornflour, cinnamon, pepper, and lemon juice,
taking care not to mash the fruit.

3 For the crumble, combine the flour, sugar, vanilla,
and salt in a mixing bowl. Gently rub in the butter
or margarine with your fingertips until the mixture
resembles breadcrumbs.

4 Transfer the fruit mixture to the baking dish, then
sprinkle the crumble evenly over the top. Bake for
about 40 minutes until the topping is golden brown and
the fruit juices are bubbling. Serve warm or at room
temperature.

Topping

You can mix the ingredients
for the crumble topping in
a food processor instead
of rubbing in the butter or
margarine by hand.

DESSERTS

Serves **4** | Prep time: **10 mins** | Cooking time: **45 mins**

KHEER

This milk pudding contains grains, milk, ghee, and almonds, making it a good dish for increasing ojas. It is beneficial for all constitutions, but those eating for kapha should eat only half a portion.

INGREDIENTS

8 tbsp white Basmati rice

400ml (14fl oz) milk by dosha
- **VATA** & **PITTA** full-fat milk
- **KAPHA** skimmed milk

1 tsp ground cardamom

4 tbsp dates, pitted and chopped

8 tbsp agave syrup or rice syrup

2 tbsp rosewater

4 tbsp ghee or coconut oil
- **KAPHA** 2 tbsp

4 tbsp blanched almonds, peeled and chopped
- **KAPHA** 2 tbsp

4 tbsp desiccated coconut

pinch of freshly ground black pepper (optional)

1 Put the rice in a heavy-based saucepan, pour in 300ml (10fl oz) of water, and bring to the boil. Cover and simmer on a low heat for 25 minutes or until the rice turns soft and has absorbed all the water.

2 Mash the cooked rice with a potato masher or a wooden spoon. Add the milk and the cardamom and bring to the boil. Simmer on a low heat for another 5 minutes, stirring constantly to prevent the mixture burning on the bottom of the pan. Remove from the heat and add in the dates, sweetener, and rosewater.

3 Fry the blanched almonds in the ghee or oil until they are golden brown, then add the coconut. If cooking for kapha dosha, add a pinch of black pepper as well. The coconut will turn golden brown very quickly, so be careful to not burn it. Add the nut mixture to the milk pudding and serve.

Soothing

Sweetened rice cooked with milk and sugar is described in the ancient yoga scripture *Mahabharata* as "the best of all foods". It has a soothing effect on the mind.

Serves **4** | Prep time: **3 mins**

LASSI

This cooling, refreshing drink contains sweet syrup and sour yogurt. Vata is pacified by the sweet and sour taste, pitta is pacified by the sweet taste, and kapha is pacified by the use of honey as a sweetener.

INGREDIENTS

300g (10oz) yogurt by dosha
- **VATA** & **PITTA** full-fat yogurt
- **KAPHA** low-fat yogurt

4 tbsp syrup by dosha
- **VATA** & **PITTA** agave syrup
- **KAPHA** raw honey

1 tsp ground cardamom

4 tbsp rosewater, or to taste

1 Put the yogurt, syrup or honey, cardamom, and rosewater into a food processor with 600ml (1 pint) of water and whizz until smooth; alternatively, use a hand-held blender to combine the ingredients until frothy. Pour into tall glasses and serve immediately.

Whisk

If you don't have a food processor or blender you can use a whisk to make the lassi.

YOGA

ASANAS, PRANAYAMA, AND RELAXATION

"Health is wealth, peace of mind is happiness, yoga shows the way."

SWAMI VISHNUDEVANANDA

AYURVEDA AND YOGA

Tracing their origin back to the oldest Indian scriptures, the vedas, Ayurveda and yoga are sister sciences. If yoga is performed correctly, it will help people of all doshas improve their physical and mental health.

The three aspects of yoga

A lot of people associate yoga mostly with the different asanas (yoga poses), but each pose is supported by rhythmic breathing to control energy levels (pranayama), and short periods of relaxation. While performing an asana, one must be simultaneously trying to achieve posture, breath control, and relaxation. This is something that comes with time and practice.

PRANAYAMA

Controlling the breath allows prana (life energy) to be stored and released from the solar plexus. This revitalizes the body and mind when performed before, during, and after asanas. Throughout the session, focus on the breath to reduce fatigue and boost oxygen supply.

Breath control *is important to aid movement and recharge the muscles.*

HATHA AND RAJA YOGA

These two systems are the most commonly practised worldwide. They are based on an understanding of the body and mind as vehicles of pure consciousness.

Hatha yoga, covered in this chapter, focuses on asanas, pranayama, and relaxation to unblock and channel prana (life energy).

Raja yoga, covered in the next chapter, emphasizes the mental control of prana through visualization, positive thinking, concentration, and meditation.

ASANAS

Performing the asanas (yoga poses) keeps the joints, muscles, ligaments, tendons, and other moving parts of the body healthy, increasing circulation and flexibility. They also energize all of the body systems, providing an internally orientated, non-competitive, and meditative exercise routine, while promoting an inner sense of calm.

The tree asana *is one of 12 poses featured in this chapter.*

Yoga and the doshas

The asana, pranayama, and relaxation exercises are the same for people of all constitutions, and a balanced approach to these aspects of yoga will naturally enhance the balance of all three doshas. However, the experience of performing the exercises will vary depending on a person's constitution. Look out for dosha boxes (see below) to learn how someone of your constitution might approach each exercise.

> *"A balanced approach to yoga will help stabilize all three doshas."*

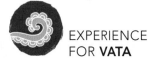

EXPERIENCE FOR **VATA**

Movement comes easily to the vata body, so practising the asanas is often pleasant. Moving slowly and holding poses can prove difficult.

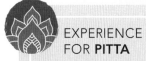

EXPERIENCE FOR **PITTA**

Those with an ambitious pitta nature should direct their focus towards the simultaneous control of breathing, posture, and relaxation.

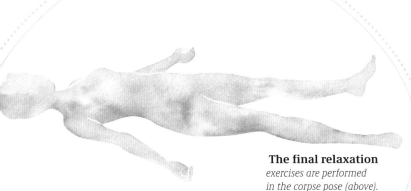

The final relaxation
exercises are performed in the corpse pose (above).

EXPERIENCE FOR **KAPHA**

The kapha body is often slow to get started during a workout, but it has good strength, patience, and endurance once it does.

RELAXATION

Even when trying to rest, many people expend a lot of energy through tension. During complete relaxation, there is little or no energy being consumed – only enough to maintain metabolic function. Short periods of rest are taken between the asanas, while longer relaxation exercises are performed as the final element of the session.

YOUR **YOGA SESSION**

This chapter follows a yoga session from start to finish. The session is the same for all constitutions. Depending on your experience, use the beginner or intermediate tips to improve your practice.

BEFORE **YOUR SESSION**
- **You will need** a yoga mat and a cushion for pranayama. You may want a blanket to stay warm during final relaxation.
- **Do not eat** for 2–3 hours before.
- **It is advised** to take a shower or bath before, but not after, practice.

1 Pranayama and warm up

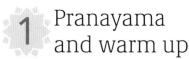

> **TIME:** about 20 minutes

Breathing and stretching exercises prepare your body for entering, holding, and releasing the asanas.

BEGINNER TIPS

- **Never strain your breath** during breathing exercises. If you feel your breath starting to strain, hold it for a shorter time than given or reduce the number of breaths in the exercise.
- **If you find** yourself discomforted, substitute the rest of the breathing exercises with slow abdominal breathing.

INTERMEDIATE TIPS

- **As you become** more comfortable with the breathing exercises, use them to focus on your awareness of your body.
- **Relax with** long exhalations and recharge with long inhalations.
- **When comfortable,** settle your mind on your third eye (see p.176).

PRANAYAMA EXERCISES

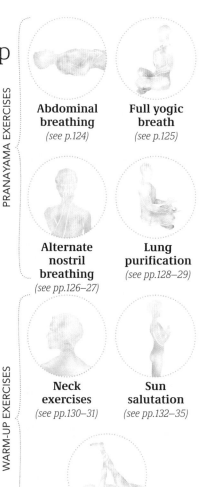

Abdominal breathing
(see p.124)

Full yogic breath
(see p.125)

Alternate nostril breathing
(see pp.126–27)

Lung purification
(see pp.128–29)

WARM-UP EXERCISES

Neck exercises
(see pp.130–31)

Sun salutation
(see pp.132–35)

Single leg lift
(see pp.136–37)

2 Asana practice

> **TIME:** about 35 minutes

These poses make up the core of the session. Make sure you relax for 1–2 minutes between each asana before moving on.

BEGINNER TIPS

- **Observe how** easy you find posture, rhythmic breathing, and relaxation while holding each asana.
- **If an asana** becomes easier, increase the time you hold it.
- **If your** breathing becomes faster and you become tense, reduce the time you hold an asana.

INTERMEDIATE TIPS

- **As you become comfortable** with each asana, focus on slowly entering and leaving it with precision and grace.
- **Keep a count** of the length of your breaths during the entire yoga session to improve your concentration.
- **Observe how** the combined effort of your arms and legs support your spine position.

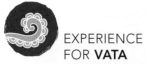

EXPERIENCE FOR **VATA**

The sun salutation aids the vata body with breath control, while relaxation between asanas prevents overexertion.

EXPERIENCE FOR **PITTA**

Pranayama deepens the breath, allowing the pitta body to safely expand stretches during the sun salutation and asanas.

EXPERIENCE FOR **KAPHA**

Those of a kapha nature will find their motivation increases with each asana as blood circulation and prana increases.

Shoulderstand
(see pp.138–39)

Plough
(see pp.140–41)

Fish
(see pp.142–43)

3 Final relaxation

Active relaxation
(see pp.160–61)

⌛ **TIME:** about 20 minutes

Use these exercises to find a state of complete relaxation, recharging your body after the exertion of the asanas.

BEGINNER TIPS

- **At first,** allow more time for active relaxation than for autosuggestion.
- **As you feel** more comfortable in the corpse pose (used for relaxation), start to bring in autosuggestion techniques.
- **Observe how** the release of tension increases your vital energy.

Relaxing with autosuggestion
(see pp.162–63)

INTERMEDIATE TIPS

- **As you** become comfortable with autosuggestion, approach this final relaxation as a detached observer.
- **Actualize the** power of each thought command.
- **Remain awake** and aware using conscious breathing.

Sitting forward bend
(see pp.144–45)

Inclined plane
(see pp.146–47)

Cobra
(see pp.148–49)

Child's pose
(see p.150)

Camel
(see p.151)

Tree
(see pp.152–53)

Crow
(see pp.154–55)

Spinal twist
(see pp.156–57)

Triangle
(see pp.158–59)

THE **YOGIC** BREATH

Pranayama (energy control through breathing) is one of the three key aspects of yoga. Practise the breathing exercises on the following pages at the beginning of each session.

PHYSICAL **BENEFITS**

- **Improves movement** of oxygen and carbon dioxide throughout the body.
- **Relaxes and recharges** the nervous system.

EXPERIENCE FOR **VATA**

The smaller vata rib cage and sensitive nervous system both benefit from the expansion provided by abdominal breathing.

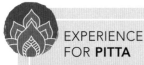

EXPERIENCE FOR **PITTA**

The greater sensory awareness provided by abdominal breathing is beneficial for balancing the overachieving pitta nature.

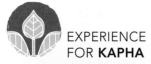

EXPERIENCE FOR **KAPHA**

The compact kapha frame will enjoy the free abdominal movement without any physical or mental restrictions.

Abdominal breathing

This technique is important for pranayama as it draws air into the lowest (and largest) part of the lungs. Completely relax your abdominal muscles so your diaphragm can move freely.

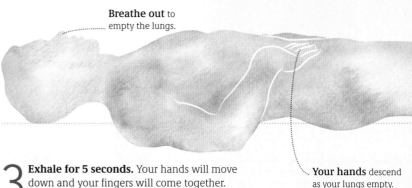

Notice your hands rising as your lungs fill with air.

Breathe in to fill the lungs.

1 **Lie on your back,** palms on your abdomen and fingers apart. As you breathe, feel the movement between your first rib, your navel, and your hips.

2 **Inhale for 5 seconds.** Pay attention to how your hands rise and your fingers draw apart as your abdomen expands.

Breathe out to empty the lungs.

3 **Exhale for 5 seconds.** Your hands will move down and your fingers will come together. Repeat these steps for 2 minutes.

Your hands descend as your lungs empty.

Full yogic breath

This technique uses all of your respiratory muscles, improving your muscle strength when moving into, holding, and releasing asanas. Performing it between asanas quickly replenishes the oxygen levels in the blood – you might want to try a few full yogic breaths at work to boost your energy levels.

1 **Sit in a** comfortable, cross-legged position. Place one hand on your chest and the other on your abdomen. As you inhale, gradually expand your abdomen, raise and open your rib cage, and lift your collar bones.

Feel your upper hand rise as you breathe in.

Keep your shoulders relaxed as you breathe in.

You may want to sit on a cushion to improve your spine alignment and release tension from your knees.

2 **Start exhaling by** relaxing the abdomen, then lower the rib cage, and, finally, slightly contract the abdomen to empty the lungs. Repeat the steps for about 2 minutes.

Keep your head, neck, and spine aligned.

Always start exhaling from the abdomen.

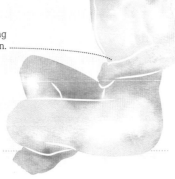

THE **SOLAR PLEXUS**

This network of nerves located behind the stomach, the solar plexus, is said to function without voluntary control. However, the yogis have discovered that conscious, slow, rhythmical abdominal breathing does have a direct effect on the solar plexus, helping it to balance its three major functions:

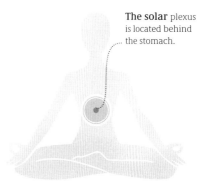

The solar plexus is located behind the stomach.

- **When stimulated,** the solar plexus brings sensory awareness to the entire abdominal area. This sensitivity can be used to discover hidden tensions in the body.
- **Abdominal breathing** generates a natural defence against stress, especially when it is combined with alternate nostril breathing (see pp.126–27) or lung purification (see pp.128–29).
- **Finally, nerve impulses** created in the solar plexus by slow abdominal exhalations during breathing, asanas, and relaxation exercises stimulate "rest and repair" throughout the body.

NOW MOVE ON TO
ALTERNATE NOSTRIL BREATHING

ALTERNATE NOSTRIL **BREATHING**

Alternate nostril breathing requires deep inhalation, prolonged breath retention, and deep exhalation. The flow of air alternates between both nostrils during the exercise.

PHYSICAL **BENEFITS**

- **Long inhalations** increase oxygen levels in the blood.
- **Long exhalations** allow for good elimination of carbon dioxide.
- **Breath retention** strengthens the nervous system.

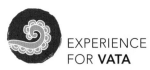

EXPERIENCE FOR **VATA**

The deep inhalation and breath holding are especially beneficial for developing and expanding vata's lung capacity.

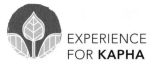

EXPERIENCE FOR **PITTA**

The prolonged exhalation promotes both relaxation and an increase in prana. This is a new experience for those of a pitta nature.

EXPERIENCE FOR **KAPHA**

The natural kapha endurance and patience will mean they simply enjoy performing alternate nostril breathing.

Simple alternate nostril breathing

Attempt this exercise first when practising alternate nostril breathing. Use the mudra hand position, shown in step 1, to close your nostrils. Practise ten rounds of the steps. Gradually increase the inhalation-to-exhalation ratio as you feel comfortable doing so, moving on from 5 seconds to 10 seconds, then 6 seconds to 12 seconds, and finally 7 seconds to 14 seconds.

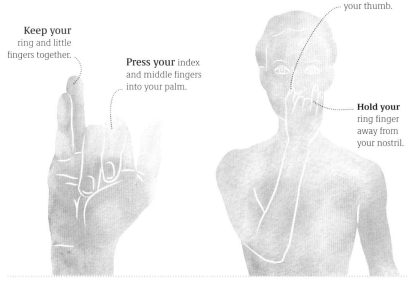

Keep your ring and little fingers together.

Press your index and middle fingers into your palm.

Press your nostril closed with the pad of your thumb.

Hold your ring finger away from your nostril.

1 **Bend your right** arm at the elbow and bring your hand close to your nose. Then, bend your index and middle fingers, gently pressing them against the palm of your hand.

2 **Closing your right** nostril with your thumb, inhale through your left nostril for 4 seconds. Close your left nostril with your ring finger, open your right nostril, and exhale for 8 seconds.

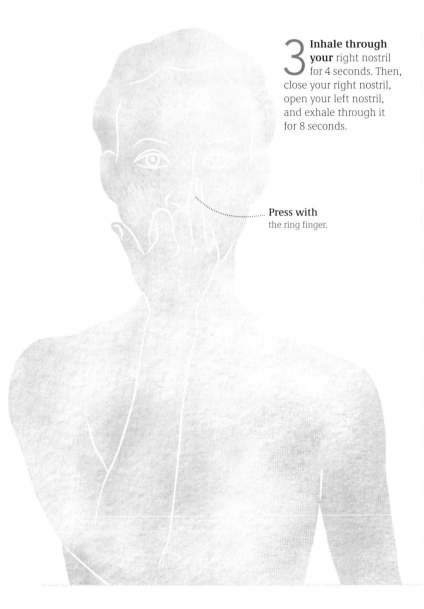

"Pranayama harmonizes the nerves and awakens the life force."

SWAMI SIVANANDA

3 **Inhale through your** right nostril for 4 seconds. Then, close your right nostril, open your left nostril, and exhale through it for 8 seconds.

Press with
the ring finger.

INTERMEDIATE VARIATION

Once you have mastered the 7:14 ratio of the simple alternate nostril breathing, try adding breath retention.

1 **Inhale through your** left nostril for 4 seconds, close the nostril, hold your breath for 8 seconds, then exhale through your right nostril for 8 seconds.

2 **Inhale through your** right nostril for 4 seconds, hold your breath for 8 seconds and exhale through your left nostril for 8 seconds.

3 **Practise up to** ten rounds. Increase the inhalation-to-retention-to-exhalation ratio to 5:10:10, then to 6:12:12, and finally to 7:14:14.

ADVANCED VARIATION

As you feel more comfortable performing a breath retention of 14 seconds, try holding your breath for a longer period.

1 **Inhale through your** left nostril for 4 seconds, hold your breath for 16 seconds, and then exhale through your right nostril for 8 seconds.

2 **Inhale through your** right nostril for 4 seconds, hold your breath for 16 seconds, and then exhale through your left nostril for 8 seconds.

3 **Practise up to** ten rounds. Increase the inhalation-to-retention-to-exhalation ratio to 5:20:10, then 6:24:12.

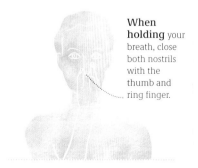

When holding your breath, close both nostrils with the thumb and ring finger.

NOW MOVE ON TO
LUNG PURIFICATION

LUNG **PURIFICATION**

Called "kapalabhati" in Sanskrit (literally "shining skull"), this process increases oxygen levels in the blood. This benefits every body system so much that, when practised regularly, the face shines.

PHYSICAL **BENEFITS**

- **Cleanses the** nasal passage, lungs, and respiratory system.
- **Increases carbon** dioxide removal and oxygen absorption.
- **Improves digestion** by massaging the abdominal organs.

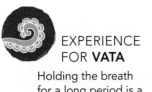

EXPERIENCE FOR **VATA**

Holding the breath for a long period is a challenge for vata, and an opportunity to expand lung capacity.

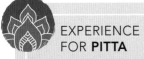

EXPERIENCE FOR **PITTA**

The pitta body can hold its breath for the longest. This results in a meditative state that balances the sharp edge of the pitta nature.

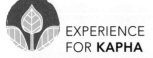

EXPERIENCE FOR **KAPHA**

The kapha body is prone to respiratory congestion. This is quickly remedied by this exercise, which gives a feeling of lightness.

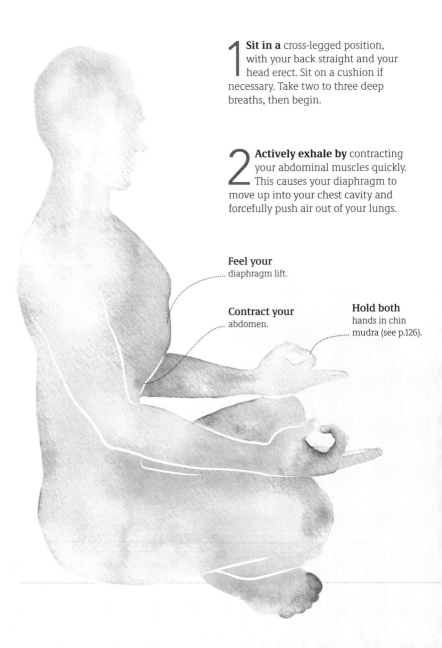

1 Sit in a cross-legged position, with your back straight and your head erect. Sit on a cushion if necessary. Take two to three deep breaths, then begin.

2 Actively exhale by contracting your abdominal muscles quickly. This causes your diaphragm to move up into your chest cavity and forcefully push air out of your lungs.

Feel your diaphragm lift.

Contract your abdomen.

Hold both hands in chin mudra (see p.126).

"While the act of pranayama is physical, the effect is to make the mind calm, lucid, and steady."

SWAMI VISHNUDEVANANDA

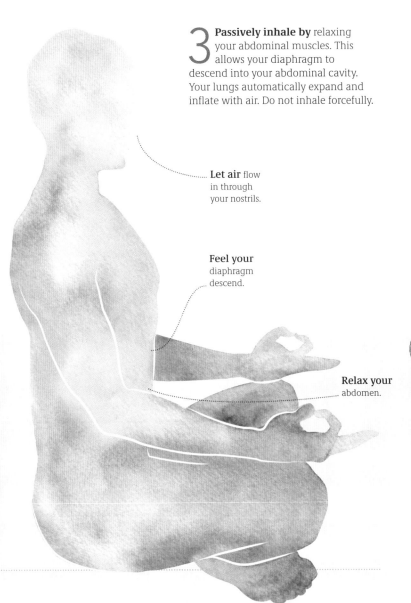

3 **Passively inhale by** relaxing your abdominal muscles. This allows your diaphragm to descend into your abdominal cavity. Your lungs automatically expand and inflate with air. Do not inhale forcefully.

Let air flow in through your nostrils.

Feel your diaphragm descend.

Relax your abdomen.

4 **Repeat steps** 2 and 3 quickly in a pumping action. Perform 20–30 exhalations and 20–30 inhalations to complete a round, ending on an exhalation. Take two deep breaths, then hold your breath for 30–60 seconds. Perform three rounds. As your capacity increases, gradually lengthen the exercise to five rounds of 50–100 cycles.

IMPORTANT NOTE

Lung purification should not be practised if you have any abdominal pain or cramping. Do not practise it late in the evening, since it activates the nervous system and may prevent you from falling asleep.

NOW MOVE ON TO
NECK EXERCISES

NECK EXERCISES

These exercises warm up your neck, shoulders, and upper back areas, aiming to reduce tension and stress. While performing them, move only your head and neck, and not your back and shoulders.

PHYSICAL BENEFITS

- **Warms up** neck and shoulders.
- **Helps to** relieve tension in the neck and upper back area.
- **Improves neck** alignment, improving physical and mental wellbeing.

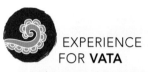

EXPERIENCE FOR VATA

These simple movements will help the vata body shift into the slow-motion mode of movement required for the asanas.

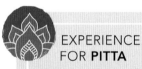

EXPERIENCE FOR PITTA

Those of a pitta nature should not exaggerate the movements too much, as these exercises are only intended to relax the neck.

1 **Keeping your back** straight, slowly allow your head to move forward and down until your chin is resting on your chest. Relax in this position. Feel as though your head is very heavy.

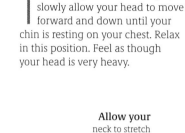

Allow your neck to stretch without straining.

Rest your chin on your chest.

2 **Lift your head** up and lower it backwards, as if trying to put the back of your head on to your spine. Repeat the first two steps six to ten times.

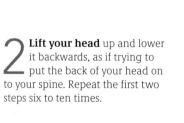

Tilt your head all the way back.

Reduce the angle of your head position if you feel any dizziness or discomfort.

EXPERIENCE FOR KAPHA

The kapha body and mind will enjoy these easy movements, and be encouraged to explore the next steps of the session.

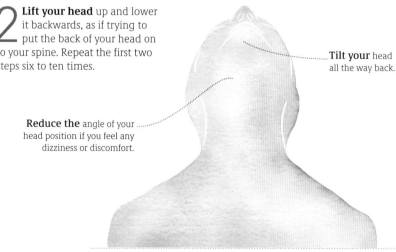

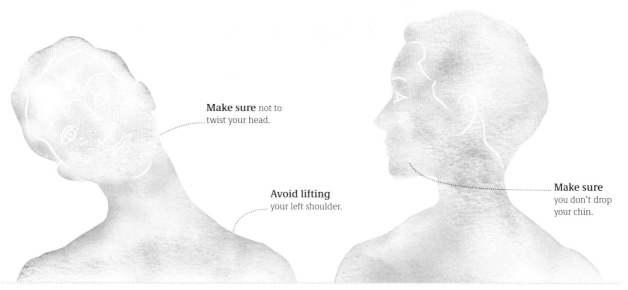

Make sure not to twist your head.

Avoid lifting your left shoulder.

Make sure you don't drop your chin.

3 **Keeping both shoulders** down, tilt your head to the right, as if trying to bring your ear down to your shoulder. Then stretch to the left side. Repeat this step five to ten times.

4 **Keeping your body** still, turn your head so that your chin is over your right shoulder. Feel the stretch on your left side, then turn your head over your left shoulder. Repeat six to ten times.

5 **Rotate your neck** and head clockwise two to three times – head forward, chin to chest, right ear to right shoulder, head back, left ear to left shoulder, head forward. Then repeat the rotation anti-clockwise two to three times.

"May all beings everywhere be free and happy."

UNIVERSAL INDIAN PRAYER

Make sure to tilt your head and not turn it.

NOW MOVE ON TO
SUN SALUTATION

SUN **SALUTATION**

Begin your session with this excellent warm-up exercise that improves the muscle efficiency for the other asanas. Perform four to six cycles, then rest in corpse pose (see pp.160–61).

PHYSICAL **BENEFITS**

- **Stretches dozens** of muscles throughout the body.
- **Quickly warms** up the body, improving muscle flexibility.
- **Regulates the** breathing and increases lung capacity.

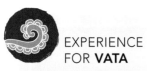

EXPERIENCE FOR **VATA**

These gently flowing movements are attractive to those of a vata nature, as they have the desire to be constantly moving.

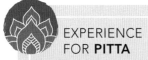

EXPERIENCE FOR **PITTA**

This exercise suits the balanced pitta nature because it is a systematic workout for both muscle length and strength.

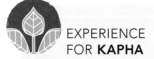

EXPERIENCE FOR **KAPHA**

Movement is not in kapha's nature, so this exercise may be resisted initially. However, it will bring an enjoyable tension release.

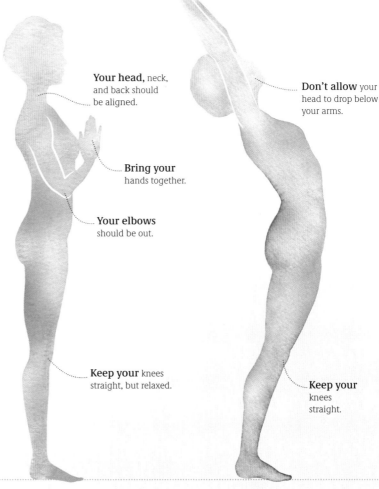

Your head, neck, and back should be aligned.

Bring your hands together.

Your elbows should be out.

Keep your knees straight, but relaxed.

Don't allow your head to drop below your arms.

Keep your knees straight.

1 Stand with your head and body straight but relaxed, and your arms relaxed by your sides. Inhale deeply, and then begin. Exhale, bring your hands together at the centre of your chest with your palms flat against each other. Keep your head upright.

2 Inhale, stretch your arms up over your head and arch your body backwards, stretching your chest and abdomen. Your arms should finish the movement alongside your ears. Keep your knees and elbows straight, and your hips arched slightly forwards.

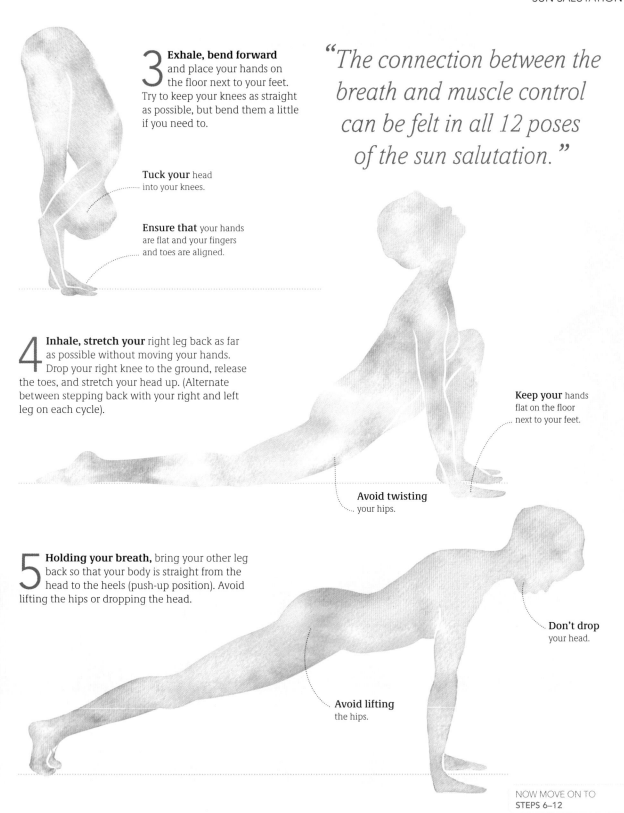

3 **Exhale, bend forward** and place your hands on the floor next to your feet. Try to keep your knees as straight as possible, but bend them a little if you need to.

Tuck your head into your knees.

Ensure that your hands are flat and your fingers and toes are aligned.

"The connection between the breath and muscle control can be felt in all 12 poses of the sun salutation."

4 **Inhale, stretch your** right leg back as far as possible without moving your hands. Drop your right knee to the ground, release the toes, and stretch your head up. (Alternate between stepping back with your right and left leg on each cycle).

Keep your hands flat on the floor next to your feet.

Avoid twisting your hips.

5 **Holding your breath,** bring your other leg back so that your body is straight from the head to the heels (push-up position). Avoid lifting the hips or dropping the head.

Don't drop your head.

Avoid lifting the hips.

NOW MOVE ON TO
STEPS 6–12

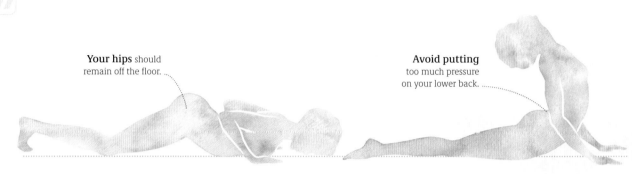

Your hips should remain off the floor.

Avoid putting too much pressure on your lower back.

6 **Exhale, and without** rocking backwards, lower your knees, chest, and forehead to the floor. Keep your hips and abdomen raised slightly, and your toes curled under.

7 **Inhale, lower your** hips to the mat, arch your head and upper spine backwards, and look up. Your elbows should be slightly bent, and your shoulders relaxed and away from your ears.

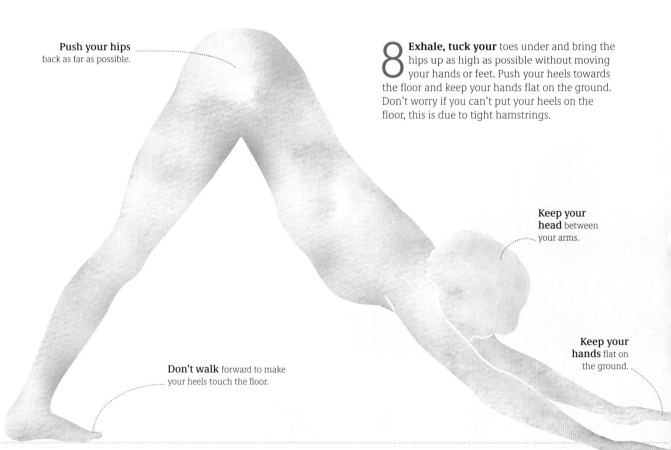

Push your hips back as far as possible.

8 **Exhale, tuck your** toes under and bring the hips up as high as possible without moving your hands or feet. Push your heels towards the floor and keep your hands flat on the ground. Don't worry if you can't put your heels on the floor, this is due to tight hamstrings.

Keep your head between your arms.

Keep your hands flat on the ground.

Don't walk forward to make your heels touch the floor.

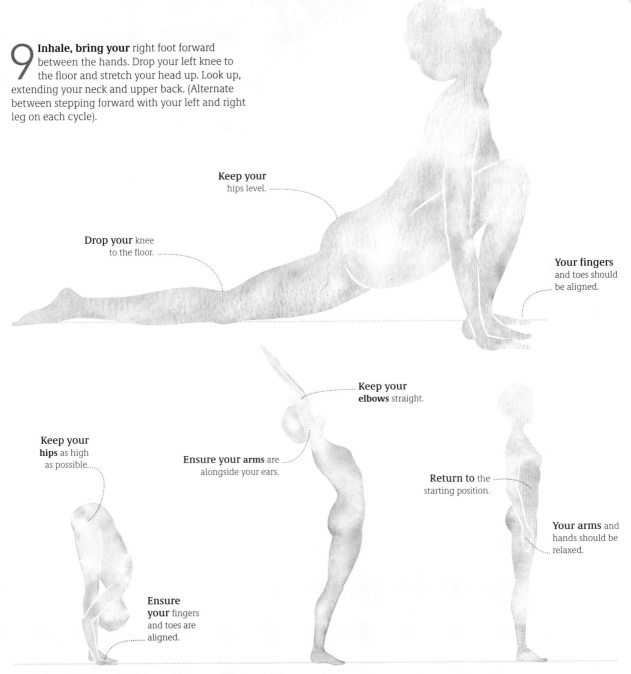

9 **Inhale, bring your** right foot forward between the hands. Drop your left knee to the floor and stretch your head up. Look up, extending your neck and upper back. (Alternate between stepping forward with your left and right leg on each cycle).

Keep your hips level.

Drop your knee to the floor.

Your fingers and toes should be aligned.

Keep your elbows straight.

Keep your hips as high as possible.

Ensure your arms are alongside your ears.

Return to the starting position.

Your arms and hands should be relaxed.

Ensure your fingers and toes are aligned.

10 **Exhale, keeping your** hands in place, bring your left foot forward so it is next to your right foot. Straighten both legs as much as possible and bend down so that your head tucks into your knees (like step 3).

11 **Inhale, stretch up** and arch backwards (the same as step 2). Make sure that you don't drop your head below your arms, as this causes undue pressure on your back. Keep your knees straight.

12 **Exhale, bring your** arms forward and down alongside your body, returning your body to the starting position. Relax for a moment, and take a deep breath so that you are ready to begin the next cycle.

NOW MOVE ON TO
SINGLE LEG LIFT

SINGLE **LEG LIFT**

This exercise will gently help you to overcome stiffness in your calves and hamstrings, preparing you for the forward bending asanas that stretch all of the muscles at the back of your body.

PHYSICAL **BENEFITS**

- **Improves flexibility** of, and relieves tension in, the calf and hamstring muscles.
- **Strengthens the** abdominal and lower back muscles.

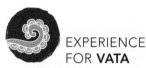

EXPERIENCE FOR **VATA**

The vata body has a temperamental and excitable nervous system that will be soothed by this slow hamstring stretch.

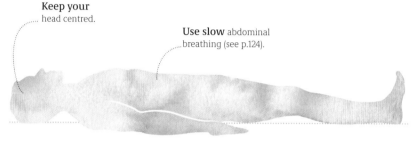

Keep your head centred.

Use slow abdominal breathing (see p.124).

1 **Lie on your** back with your feet together and place your hands palms down on the floor by your sides.

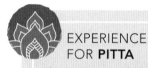

EXPERIENCE FOR **PITTA**

The pitta nature has a drive for movement and perfection that will be satisfied by stretching out the hamstrings in this way.

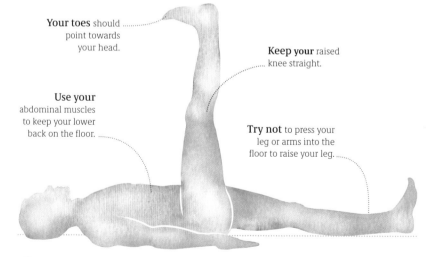

Your toes should point towards your head.

Keep your raised knee straight.

Use your abdominal muscles to keep your lower back on the floor.

Try not to press your leg or arms into the floor to raise your leg.

2 **Inhale, bring your** right leg perpendicular to the floor. Exhale, lower your raised leg, ensuring that your other leg remains straight. Repeat with your left leg. Do three to five sets and, on the last set of leg raises, follow step 3.

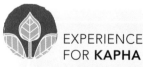

EXPERIENCE FOR **KAPHA**

Those of a kapha nature will enjoy the feeling of lightness in the legs provided by this exercise.

WORKING TOWARDS
SINGLE LEG LIFT

If you find the exercise too strenuous for your back, bend your other knee before raising your leg.

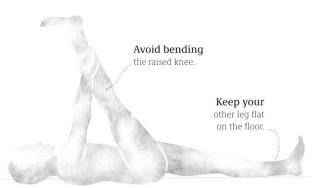

Bend your other knee to reduce the intensity of the stretch.

Avoid bending the raised knee.

Keep your other leg flat on the floor.

Hold your leg if you are unable to reach your foot.

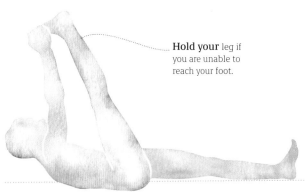

3 **Inhale, raise your** right leg and, clasping it in both hands, pull it towards you, keeping your head down. Hold the position for a few breaths.

4 **Exhale, now holding** your right foot in both hands, lift your back off the mat, bringing your chest and head towards your raised leg.

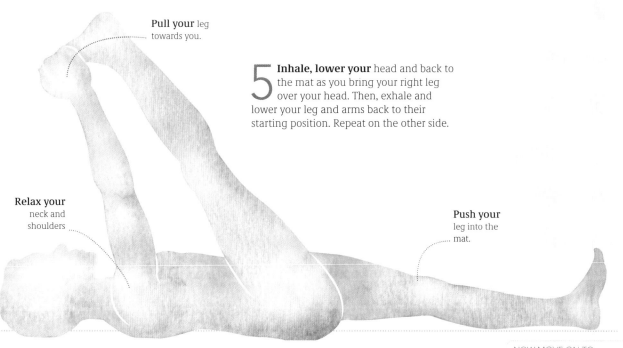

Pull your leg towards you.

Relax your neck and shoulders

5 **Inhale, lower your** head and back to the mat as you bring your right leg over your head. Then, exhale and lower your leg and arms back to their starting position. Repeat on the other side.

Push your leg into the mat.

NOW MOVE ON TO
SHOULDERSTAND

SHOULDERSTAND

This is the first of two inverted asanas performed in the session. Inversion is equally challenging for all three doshas. Follow shoulderstand with plough and then its counter-pose – fish.

PHYSICAL BENEFITS

- **Stretches away** stress in the shoulder and neck area.
- **Tones and** revitalizes the thyroid and parathyroid glands.
- **Strengthens the** heartbeat and improves bloodflow to the brain.

EXPERIENCE FOR **VATA**

Those with a vata nature find it difficult to stay still. This must be overcome to maintain good balance during this inversion.

EXPERIENCE FOR **PITTA**

It may take time to for those of a pitta nature to establish the unfamiliar muscular interplay required to hold the inversion.

EXPERIENCE FOR **KAPHA**

It may be difficult to raise the heavy kapha body into the inversion, but once achieved, maintaining the position will prove easier.

1 Lie flat on your back with your feet together. Stretch your arms behind your head to make sure that there is enough space. Then, keeping your back, head, and neck on the mat and your arms by the side of the body, inhale and lift your legs to a 90-degree angle.

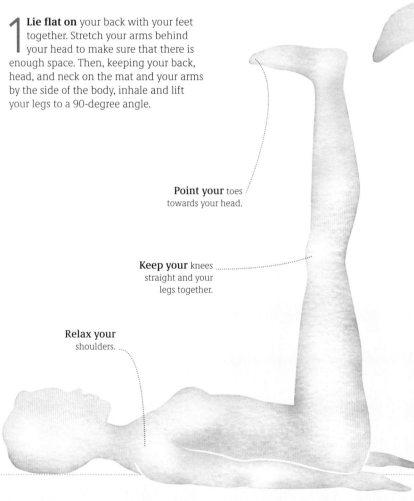

Point your toes towards your head.

Keep your knees straight and your legs together.

Relax your shoulders.

"This inverted asana creates a flow of energy that gathers in the solar plexus."

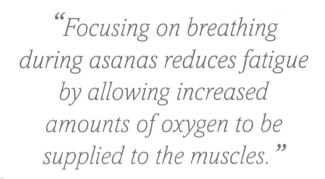

"Focusing on breathing during asanas reduces fatigue by allowing increased amounts of oxygen to be supplied to the muscles."

INTERMEDIATE VARIATION

From step 2, continue lifting your body until your legs are in a straight line with your torso. Your shoulders and elbows support your weight. From time to time, readjust your body by bringing your hands closer to your shoulders, and your elbows a bit closer to each other. To come down from the pose, return to the position in step 2, and then follow step 3.

Keep your knees straight.

Maintain a constant pressure on your back with your hands.

Relax your legs.

2 **Bring your hands** on to your buttocks and gently push the body up by walking your hands towards your lower back. Breathe slowly into your abdomen and relax your feet and legs as much as possible. Keep most of your weight on your elbows and very little on your neck and shoulders.

Your hands should support your back and point upwards.

3 **To come down** from the pose, place your hands palms down on the mat behind your back, then slowly roll down, vertebra by vertebra.

NOW MOVE ON TO
PLOUGH

PLOUGH

This is a natural continuation of the forward-bending movement of shoulderstand. If you are more experienced performing this asana, move straight into it from shoulderstand.

PHYSICAL **BENEFITS**

- **Stretches the back** muscles completely, mobilizing the spine.
- **Releases tension** in the shoulder and neck muscles.
- **Improves digestion** and combats constipation.

EXPERIENCE FOR **VATA**

Breathing in this asana can be difficult with a narrow vata ribcage. Those of a vata nature should breathe slowly and deeply before starting.

EXPERIENCE FOR **PITTA**

With over half of the body's weight on the sensitive neck muscles, those with a pitta nature should avoid ambition and apply the stretch gradually.

EXPERIENCE FOR **KAPHA**

If breathing becomes difficult, those with a kapha nature should hold plough for only a few breaths. Then rest and repeat.

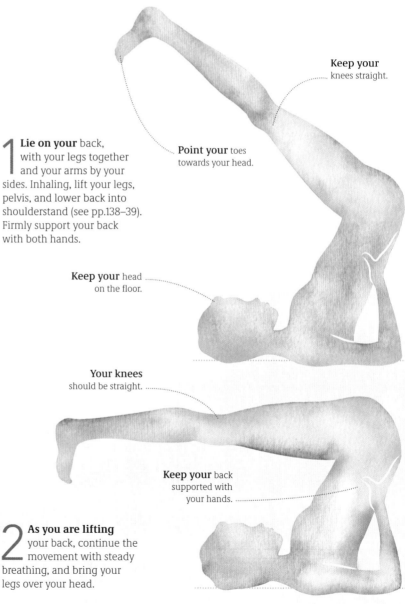

1 Lie on your back, with your legs together and your arms by your sides. Inhaling, lift your legs, pelvis, and lower back into shoulderstand (see pp.138–39). Firmly support your back with both hands.

Keep your knees straight.

Point your toes towards your head.

Keep your head on the floor.

Your knees should be straight.

Keep your back supported with your hands.

2 As you are lifting your back, continue the movement with steady breathing, and bring your legs over your head.

"The weight-bearing forward bend of plough keeps your spine supple."

INTERMEDIATE
VARIATION

If you are able to touch the ground with your feet when you are performing step 3, lower your arms to the floor behind your back to go into the full position.

Try to keep your spine straight.

Keep your arms as close to each other as possible.

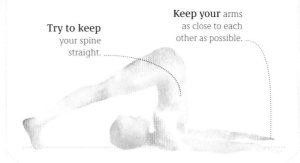

3 **Keeping your legs** straight and toes flexed, stretch your feet down towards the floor behind you. Release the pose by rolling down vertebra by vertebra, with your arms pushing against the floor for balance.

Make sure your legs are together.

Your back should still be supported with your hands.

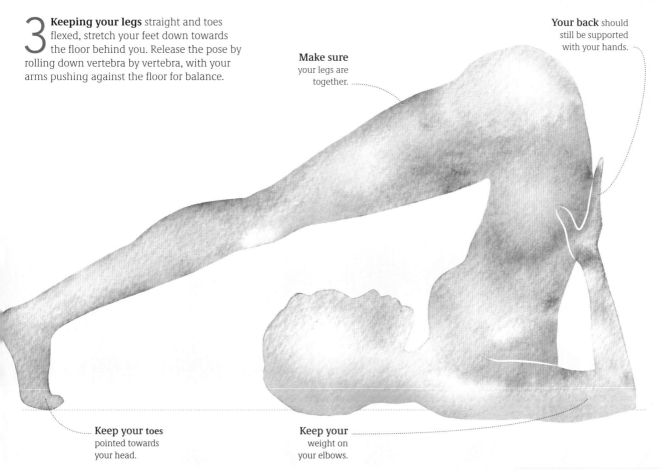

Keep your toes pointed towards your head.

Keep your weight on your elbows.

NOW MOVE ON TO
FISH

FISH

This counter-pose should follow plough. It relieves any congestion or tension which may have been caused by the previous two positions, and opens the chest for deep breathing.

PHYSICAL **BENEFITS**

- **Corrects any** tendency to hunch the shoulders.
- **Develops lung** capacity.
- **Relieves tension** and congestion in the lungs.

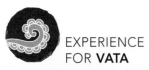

EXPERIENCE FOR **VATA**

This asana is ideal for expanding the narrow rib cage of the vata body, allowing for greater prana (vital energy) capacity.

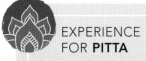

EXPERIENCE FOR **PITTA**

There is a natural limit to this stretch, which makes it ideal for slowing down and relaxing the sharp and ambitious pitta nature.

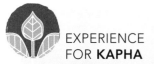

EXPERIENCE FOR **KAPHA**

The fish has a decongestant effect that can help clear any build-up of mucous – a common occurrence in the kapha body.

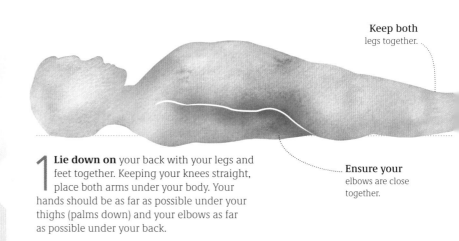

Keep both legs together.

1 **Lie down on** your back with your legs and feet together. Keeping your knees straight, place both arms under your body. Your hands should be as far as possible under your thighs (palms down) and your elbows as far as possible under your back.

Ensure your elbows are close together.

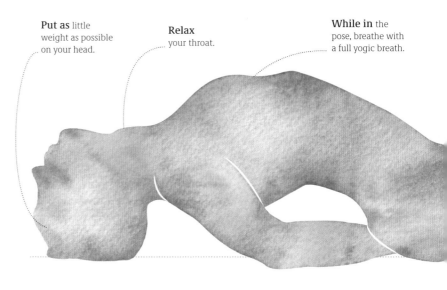

Put as little weight as possible on your head.

Relax your throat.

While in the pose, breathe with a full yogic breath.

"Observe how the asanas have a rhythmical alternation between effort and relaxation, pose and counter-pose."

NECK **STRETCH**

After fish, practise this pose to release any tension in your neck. Interlock your fingers behind your head and hold your forearms close to your ears. Then, inhale and lift your head, pushing your chin into your chest. On an exhalation, slowly lower your head back to the mat.

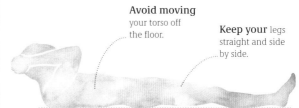

Avoid moving your torso off the floor.

Keep your legs straight and side by side.

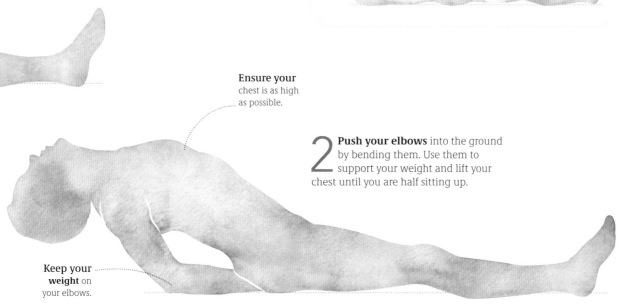

Ensure your chest is as high as possible.

2 **Push your elbows** into the ground by bending them. Use them to support your weight and lift your chest until you are half sitting up.

Keep your weight on your elbows.

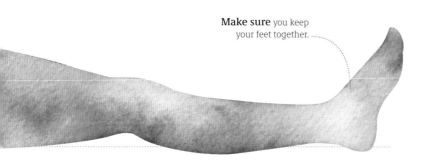

Make sure you keep your feet together.

3 **If you can** manage, slowly move your head back until it is touching the ground and your chest is expanded. To come down from the pose, lift your head slightly, lower your back to the ground, and relax in corpse pose (see pp.160–61). Slowly roll your head from side to side once or twice, then bring it back to the centre.

NOW MOVE ON TO
SITTING FORWARD BEND

SITTING **FORWARD BEND**

The sitting forward bend stretches all the muscles at the back of the body – from toe to neck – and provides an abdominal massage. Perform its counter-pose, inclined plane, afterwards.

PHYSICAL **BENEFITS**

- **Restores flexibility** to the leg and back muscles.
- **Helps to** correct an exaggerated lower back curve.
- **Tones the** digestive organs and helps to regulate the pancreas.

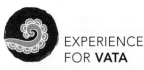

EXPERIENCE FOR **VATA**

Those of a vata nature will find that holding the forward bend will be a helpful exercise to balance their often fidgety nature.

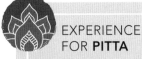

EXPERIENCE FOR **PITTA**

Athletic pitta bodies often have tight hamstrings. The deep leg stretch of the forward bend can therefore be a challenge.

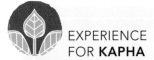

EXPERIENCE FOR **KAPHA**

This exercise is both meditative and stimulating, so will prove a rewarding experience for the stationary kapha nature.

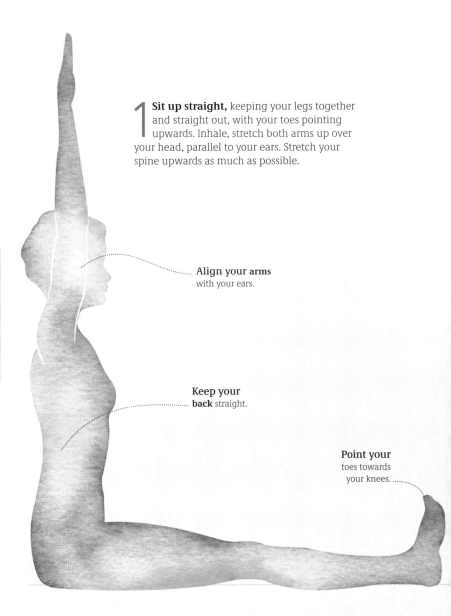

1 **Sit up straight,** keeping your legs together and straight out, with your toes pointing upwards. Inhale, stretch both arms up over your head, parallel to your ears. Stretch your spine upwards as much as possible.

Align your arms with your ears.

Keep your back straight.

Point your toes towards your knees.

2 **Retaining the stretch** and pulling the abdomen in, exhale and fold forward from the pelvis, leading with the chest and keeping your back straight.

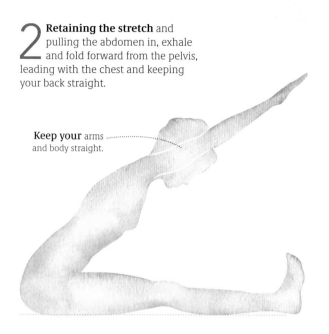

Keep your arms and body straight.

INTERMEDIATE
VARIATION

If you are comfortable in step 3, try to bring your abdomen as close to your thighs as possible. Make sure that you keep your knees as straight as possible.

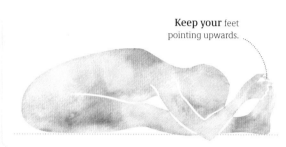

Keep your feet pointing upwards.

3 **Bend forward until** your hands reach either your shins, ankles, or feet, and stretch your head and spine forwards as much as possible. Let your elbows hang loose to release tension in your neck and shoulders. Breathe slowly and deeply. Visualize the top of your head moving towards your feet.

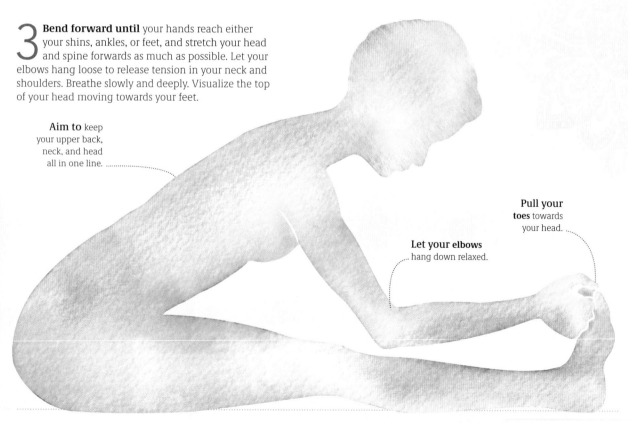

Aim to keep your upper back, neck, and head all in one line.

Pull your toes towards your head.

Let your elbows hang down relaxed.

NOW MOVE ON TO
INCLINED PLANE

INCLINED PLANE

As a counter-pose to the sitting forward bend, inclined plane contracts and strengthens the same muscles that were stretched in sitting forward bend. Relax in corpse pose afterwards.

PHYSICAL BENEFITS

- **Improves ability** to maintain balance.
- **Strengthens the** lower back, leg, and arm muscles.

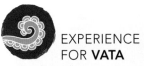

EXPERIENCE FOR **VATA**

The vata body makes inclined plane relatively easy to enter, but also makes holding the pose more difficult.

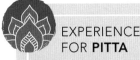

EXPERIENCE FOR **PITTA**

Those of a pitta nature should attempt to hold this pose a little longer than comfortable in order to explore their strength and willpower.

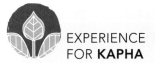

EXPERIENCE FOR **KAPHA**

Extra motivation may be needed for those of a kapha nature to get into the pose, but their naturally strong wrists should help maintain it.

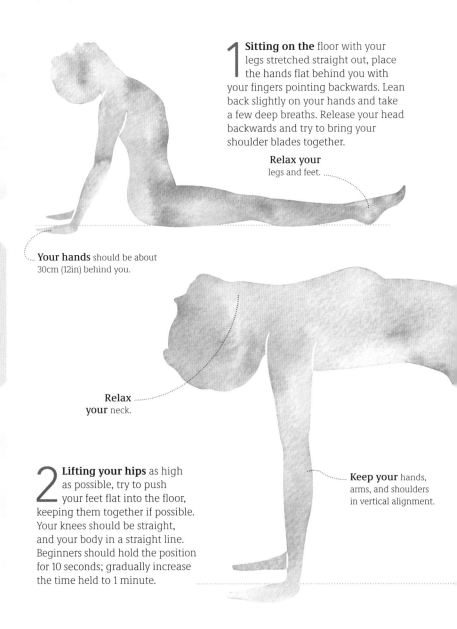

1 **Sitting on the** floor with your legs stretched straight out, place the hands flat behind you with your fingers pointing backwards. Lean back slightly on your hands and take a few deep breaths. Release your head backwards and try to bring your shoulder blades together.

Relax your legs and feet.

Your hands should be about 30cm (12in) behind you.

Relax your neck.

2 **Lifting your hips** as high as possible, try to push your feet flat into the floor, keeping them together if possible. Your knees should be straight, and your body in a straight line. Beginners should hold the position for 10 seconds; gradually increase the time held to 1 minute.

Keep your hands, arms, and shoulders in vertical alignment.

INTERMEDIATE
VARIATION

Starting from step 2, inhale and lift your left leg straight up. Exhale, and lower your leg, then repeat the action two more times. Repeat three times on the other side.

Make sure that you keep your leg straight.

Keep your hips raised.

Keep your foot flat on the mat.

Your hands and shoulders should be vertically aligned.

Your feet should be shoulder-width apart.

Arms out either side of your body.

3 **To release the position,** sit down on the ground and shake out your wrists. Stretch your arms straight out in front and slowly roll down onto your back. Relax in corpse pose (see pp.160–61).

Keep your knees straight.

"Hold the asana comfortably but firmly. This requires finely tuned muscle control."

Try to keep your feet from turning outwards.

NOW MOVE ON TO
COBRA

COBRA

Visualize the smooth, supple movement of a
snake as you slowly stretch your spine up and
back, vertebra by vertebra. Cobra should be
followed by the child's pose.

PHYSICAL **BENEFITS**

- **Rejuvenates the** nerves and
  muscles of the spine.
- **Alleviates menstrual** pains.
- **Relieves kyphosis** – excess
  curvature of the upper spine.

EXPERIENCE FOR **VATA**

Those with a vata body
should take care not to
compensate for a lack of
mobility in the upper back
by putting pressure on the
lower back.

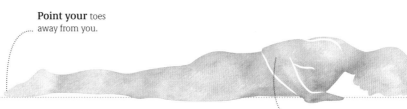

Point your toes
away from you.

1 **Lie on your** front with your legs together.
Bring the forehead to the ground. Place your
hands flat on the floor, palms downwards.
Make sure that your fingertips are in line with the
top of your shoulders.

Bend your elbows
so that they are in
towards your body and
point slightly upwards.

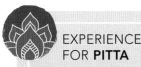

EXPERIENCE FOR **PITTA**

Those with a pitta body
have superior arm trength,
but should ensure that their
elbows remain close to the
body near the kidneys.

*"You are as young as your
spine is flexible."*

CHINESE PROVERB

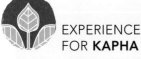

EXPERIENCE FOR **KAPHA**

For added motivation,
those of a kapha nature
should visualize how well
this asana stretches the
chest and strengthens
the upper back.

Keep your
feet together.

**Relax
your** legs.

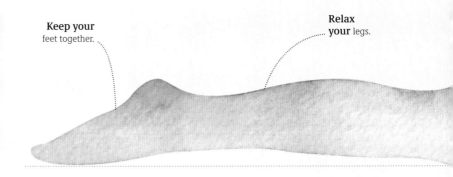

INTERMEDIATE VARIATION

After step 2, push your hands into the floor, raising your head and chest high off the ground. Feel the pressure travel downwards through your cervical, thoracic, and lumbar areas to your sacrum. Keep your hips and legs on the ground. Your elbows should remain slightly bent and your shoulders down, back, and away from your ears. Then leave the asana as described in step 2.

Extend
your neck.

Put pressure
on your hands.

Keep your
legs together.

2 **Inhale, and begin** to roll your head up and back. Curve the spine according to the strength of your back muscles. If you feel any pain, reduce the effort so that your spine bends less, remaining at a comfortable level of extension. Exhale as you roll slowly out of the posture. Uncurl your back first, keeping your head back until last and end up with your forehead on the ground.

Keep your
shoulders away
from your ears.

Avoid moving your
hips off the mat.

NOW MOVE ON TO
CHILD'S POSE

CHILD'S POSE

A counter-pose to the backward stretch of cobra, the child's pose brings a refreshing flow of blood to the brain, providing rejuvenation before you move on to the camel pose.

PHYSICAL BENEFITS

- **Stretches the** muscles in the back and around the hips.
- **Gently stretches** the spine.
- **Relaxes the** head and shoulders.

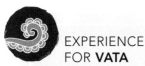

EXPERIENCE FOR **VATA**

This passive forward bend naturally increases rest and relaxation in the nervous system, so is particularly important for vata.

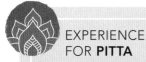

EXPERIENCE FOR **PITTA**

This asana represents humility. Those of a pitta nature should extend their exhalations and enjoy relaxing in this position.

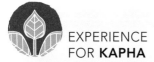

EXPERIENCE FOR **KAPHA**

Those with particularly compact kapha bodies may feel more comfortable in the asana if they keep their knees apart.

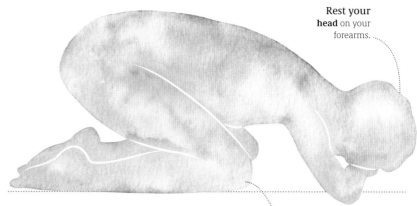

Rest your **head** on your forearms.

Keep your **knees** apart.

1 **Sit on your** heels with your knees slightly apart, lean forwards, and fold your arms on the floor in front of you, allowing your buttocks to rise off your heels. Rest your forehead on your folded arms. Breathe slowly and comfortably.

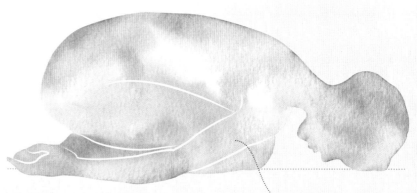

2 **Extend your arms** alongside your legs and rest your hands beside your feet, palms facing upwards. Lean forwards until your forehead touches the floor. Take at least eight deep, rhythmical breaths before progressing to camel.

Relax your **arms** beside your body.

NOW MOVE ON TO CAMEL

CAMEL

This asana stretches your chest and throat muscles, while also strengthening your hamstrings and glutes. Relax in child's pose for at least eight breaths afterwards.

PHYSICAL **BENEFITS**

- **Stretches the** throat and chest muscles.
- **Strengthens the** hamstring and glute muscles.

EXPERIENCE FOR **VATA**

Aided by their flexible nature, those with a vata body should attempt to enter and leave the asana smoothly and gracefully.

EXPERIENCE FOR **PITTA**

The pitta body has strong thighs and glute muscles to resist the powerful backward pull of gravity in this asana.

EXPERIENCE FOR **KAPHA**

This asana naturally enhances breathing. This may clear accumulated mucous, something the kapha body is prone to.

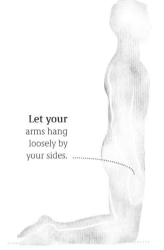

Let your arms hang loosely by your sides.

1 **Kneel on the mat** with your knees and feet hip-width apart, arms by your sides. Breathe slowly and rhythmically.

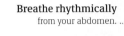

Breathe rhythmically from your abdomen.

2 **Support your back** with both hands. Inhale and slowly bend backwards, your head back first, then your shoulders and chest, and finally your lower back. Hold for up to 30 seconds, breathing slowly and rhythmically.

3 **Leave the pose** by inhaling, contracting your abdomen, and lifting your torso back up.

Keep your elbows close together.

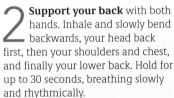
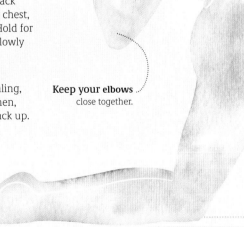

NOW MOVE ON TO TREE

TREE

Tree is the first of the balancing poses, which all require concentration and single-mindedness to maintain. To help you find your point of balance, move your weight between your heel and toes.

PHYSICAL **BENEFITS**

- **Strengthens both** the legs and feet.
- **Promotes a** strong upper back and an open rib cage.

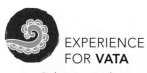

EXPERIENCE FOR **VATA**

Balancing in the tree asana naturally slows down the sometimes accelerated impulses of the vata nature.

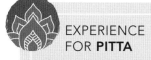

EXPERIENCE FOR **PITTA**

Those with a pitta body may find this pose too easy, so can add complexity by attempting to maintain balance with one eye closed.

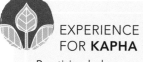

EXPERIENCE FOR **KAPHA**

Practising balance exercises brings a lightness to the body that is especially useful to the heavy kapha nature.

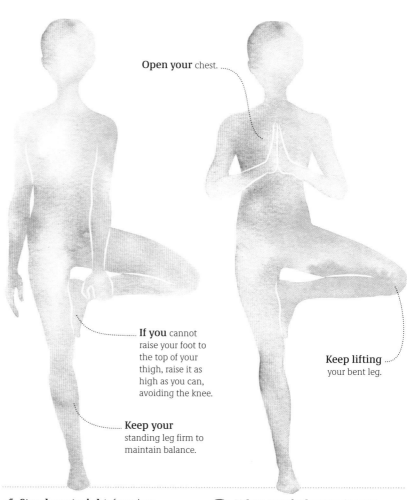

Open your chest.

If you cannot raise your foot to the top of your thigh, raise it as high as you can, avoiding the knee.

Keep your standing leg firm to maintain balance.

Keep lifting your bent leg.

1 **Stand up straight,** focusing on a spot in front of you for balance. Breathe slowly from your abdomen. Lift your left foot and place it against your right thigh.

2 **When you feel** secure in your balance, release the hold on your foot and place your hands in front of your chest, palms together. Continue breathing rhythmically.

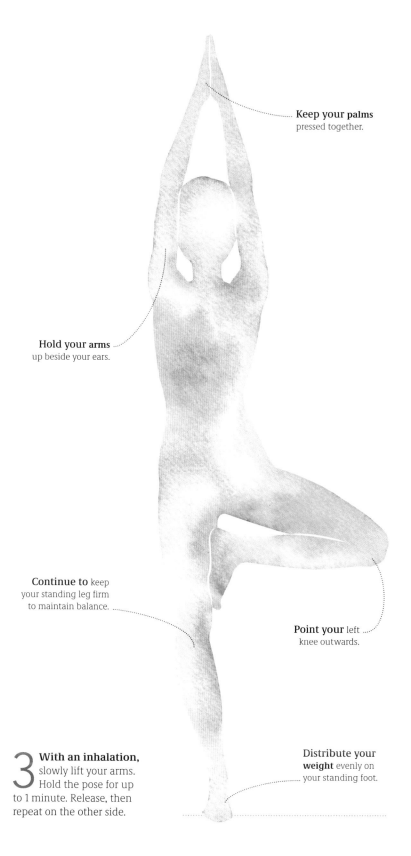

Keep your palms
pressed together.

Hold your arms
up beside your ears.

Continue to keep
your standing leg firm
to maintain balance.

Point your left
knee outwards.

3 With an inhalation,
slowly lift your arms.
Hold the pose for up
to 1 minute. Release, then
repeat on the other side.

Distribute your
weight evenly on
your standing foot.

INTERMEDIATE
VARIATION

If you are confident performing the
tree pose, try doing so in half lotus
position. Use your hands to position
your foot as with the beginner
variation, and, once comfortable, lift
your arms above your head with your
palms flat together. Hold for up to
1 minute, breathing rhythmically, then
release and repeat on the other side.

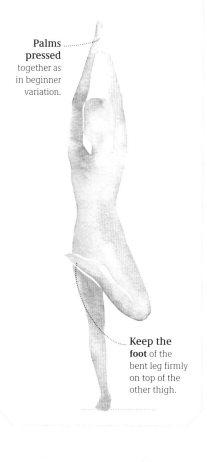

Palms
pressed
together as
in beginner
variation.

**Keep the
foot** of the
bent leg firmly
on top of the
other thigh.

NOW MOVE ON
TO **CROW**

CROW

The more challenging of the balancing asanas have long been used by yogis to build muscle strength. Crow is a perfect example of this type of strength-building exercise.

PHYSICAL BENEFITS

- **Strengthens the** arms, wrists, and shoulders.
- **Stretches the** muscles of the fingers, wrists, and forearms.
- **Improves sense** of balance.

EXPERIENCE FOR **VATA**

Those with the light and agile vata body should find this pose easy unless they have particularly delicate wrists.

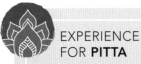

EXPERIENCE FOR **PITTA**

Those with a pitta body should try to extend their elbows a bit more and hold the asana a little longer each session.

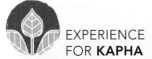

EXPERIENCE FOR **KAPHA**

With the naturally strong joints of the kapha body, those with dominant kapha may find this asana easier than they expect.

1 **Squat with your** legs and feet apart. Move your shoulders in front of your knees and your palms onto the mat in front of you. Spread your fingers wide apart, turn your wrists inwards, and bend your elbows out. Breathe slowly and rhythmically.

2 **Bring your weight** up onto your toes, raising your hips as much as possible with your knees pressed firmly against your upper arms. Look straight ahead, and continue breathing rhythmically in your abdomen.

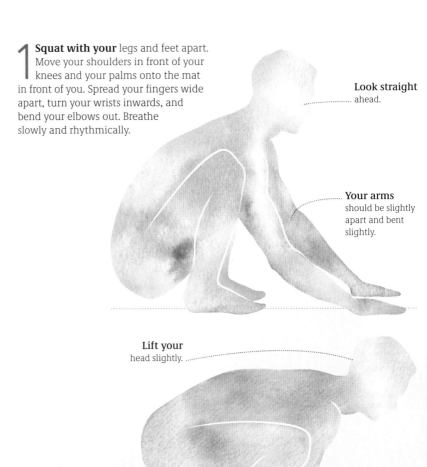

Look straight ahead.

Your arms should be slightly apart and bent slightly.

Lift your head slightly.

Bend your elbows slightly.

> *"The body follows the mind."*
>
> SWAMI SIVANANDA

INTERMEDIATE VARIATION

If your wrists are strong enough, try the full pose. Starting from step 3, inhale, hold your breath, then slowly move your weight forwards until your feet lift off of the floor. Balance for a few seconds, then exhale, and return to step 2. Once you can, hold the pose for 30 seconds while breathing rhythmically.

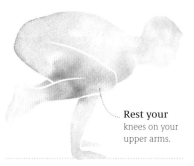

Rest your knees on your upper arms.

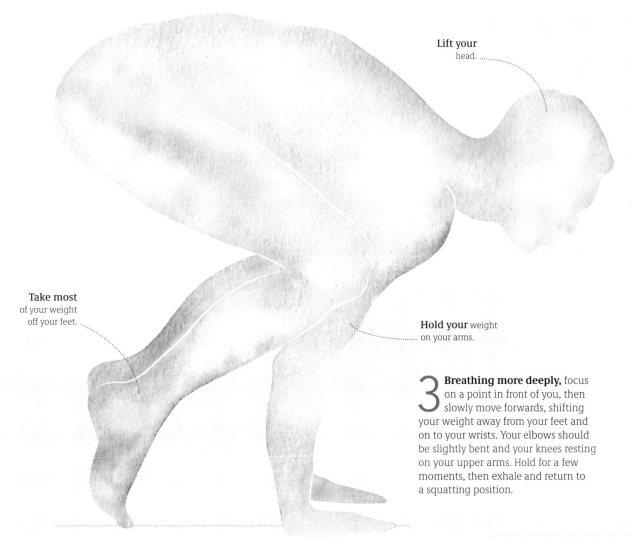

Lift your head.

Take most of your weight off your feet.

Hold your weight on your arms.

3 **Breathing more deeply,** focus on a point in front of you, then slowly move forwards, shifting your weight away from your feet and on to your wrists. Your elbows should be slightly bent and your knees resting on your upper arms. Hold for a few moments, then exhale and return to a squatting position.

NOW MOVE ON TO
SPINAL TWIST

SPINAL **TWIST**

The lumbar area of the spine does not twist easily, so you will mostly rotate the chest and neck areas. Keeping your chest open and your neck straight is the best basis for a good twist.

PHYSICAL **BENEFITS**

- **Promotes elasticity** in the spine.
- **Improves blood** circulation to the roots of the spinal nerves.
- **Helps to** relieve constipation and other digestive problems.

EXPERIENCE FOR **VATA**

The spinal twist releases pressure from the spinal nerve roots, which can help to improve the light sleep of those with dominant vata.

EXPERIENCE FOR **PITTA**

As the spinal rotation requires many types of muscles, this asana proves a delightful workout for ambitious pitta types.

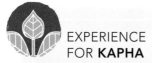

EXPERIENCE FOR **KAPHA**

The number of muscles used means that this asana requires patience to do correctly, which suits the kapha nature.

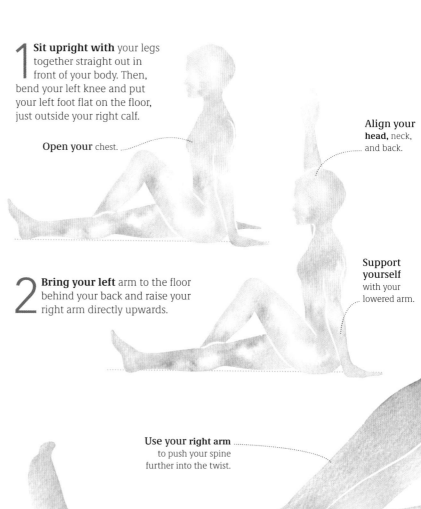

1 **Sit upright with** your legs together straight out in front of your body. Then, bend your left knee and put your left foot flat on the floor, just outside your right calf.

Open your chest.

Align your head, neck, and back.

2 **Bring your left** arm to the floor behind your back and raise your right arm directly upwards.

Support yourself with your lowered arm.

Use your right arm to push your spine further into the twist.

> *"The practice of asanas gives physical, mental, and spiritual strength."*
>
> SWAMI VISHNUDEVANANDA

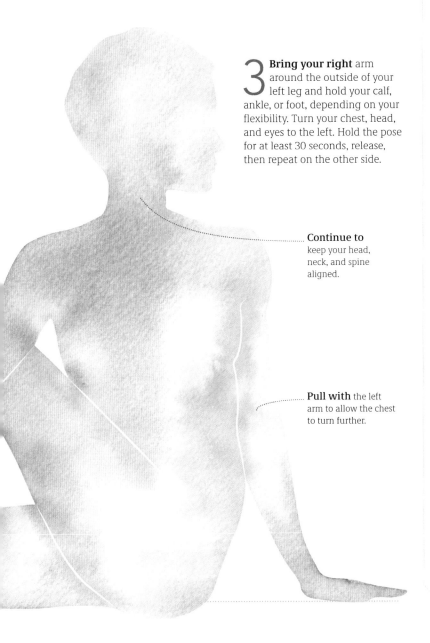

3 **Bring your right** arm around the outside of your left leg and hold your calf, ankle, or foot, depending on your flexibility. Turn your chest, head, and eyes to the left. Hold the pose for at least 30 seconds, release, then repeat on the other side.

Continue to keep your head, neck, and spine aligned.

Pull with the left arm to allow the chest to turn further.

INTERMEDIATE VARIATION

From a kneeling position, sit up on your heels and then drop your bottom to the floor to the right of your heels.

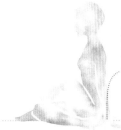

Keep your hands on the floor for stability.

1 **Raise your left leg** over your right leg, place your left foot on the mat just outside your right knee, and bring your right heel close to your buttocks.

Use this arm stretch to help lengthen the spine.

2 **With your left hand** flat on the floor behind your back, raise your right arm up.

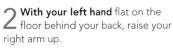

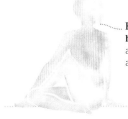

Keep the head, neck, and spine in alignment.

3 **With your right arm** over your left knee, reach around to hold your left ankle and look over your left shoulder. Breathe deeply and rhythmically.

NOW MOVE ON TO
TRIANGLE

TRIANGLE

The triangle provides a unique combination of balancing, strengthening, and stretching. It is the final asana in the session, so move on to the final relaxation part of the session when completed.

PHYSICAL **BENEFITS**

- **Tones the** spinal nerves and abdominal organs.
- **Promotes flexibility** in the legs and the hips.
- **Improves balance.**

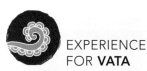

EXPERIENCE FOR **VATA**

This asana is ideal for the vata body as it requires balancing while concentrating on deep, controlled breathing.

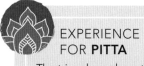

EXPERIENCE FOR **PITTA**

The triangle works out the muscles on many levels, making it particularly appealing to pitta's ambitious nature.

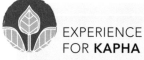

EXPERIENCE FOR **KAPHA**

The kapha body provides natural endurance to allow enjoyment of this asana's requirement for balance and strength.

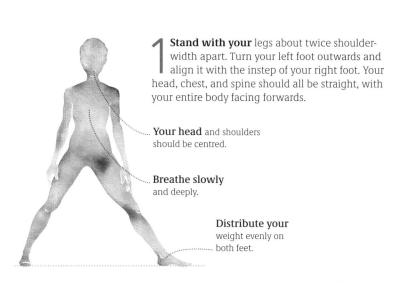

1 **Stand with your** legs about twice shoulder-width apart. Turn your left foot outwards and align it with the instep of your right foot. Your head, chest, and spine should all be straight, with your entire body facing forwards.

Your head and shoulders should be centred.

Breathe slowly and deeply.

Distribute your weight evenly on both feet.

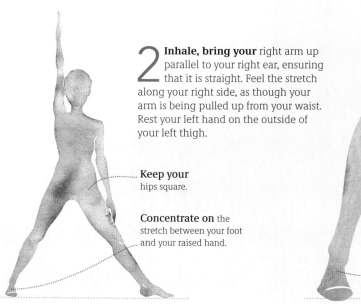

2 **Inhale, bring your** right arm up parallel to your right ear, ensuring that it is straight. Feel the stretch along your right side, as though your arm is being pulled up from your waist. Rest your left hand on the outside of your left thigh.

Keep your hips square.

Concentrate on the stretch between your foot and your raised hand.

"One gram of practice is better than tons of theory."

SWAMI SIVANANDA

WORKING TOWARDS
TRIANGLE

If you are unable to touch your foot in step 3, bend your left knee as you exhale and bend your trunk to the left. Each session, slightly reduce the bend in your knee until you are comfortable performing step 3 with a straight leg.

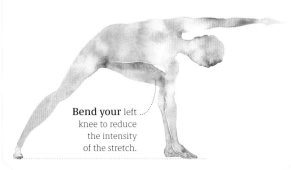

Bend your left knee to reduce the intensity of the stretch.

Your hips, trunk, and arm should be horizontally aligned.

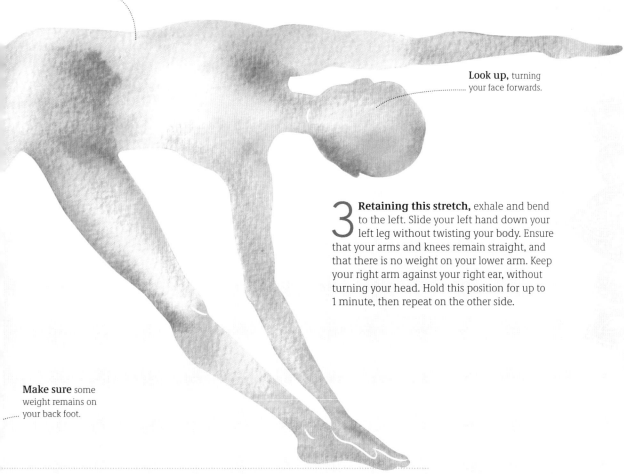

Look up, turning your face forwards.

Make sure some weight remains on your back foot.

3 **Retaining this stretch,** exhale and bend to the left. Slide your left hand down your left leg without twisting your body. Ensure that your arms and knees remain straight, and that there is no weight on your lower arm. Keep your right arm against your right ear, without turning your head. Hold this position for up to 1 minute, then repeat on the other side.

NOW MOVE ON TO
ACTIVE RELAXATION

ACTIVE RELAXATION

Short, active muscle contractions followed by a sudden and complete muscular release will remove many hidden tensions in the body. The following active relaxation exercises should be performed as the first part of the final relaxation.

Performing the corpse pose

Lie flat on your back, with your arms and legs slightly apart and relaxed. Try to align your body in a symmetrical way. Allow your back to touch the floor, and keep your legs straight, but not tensed. Relax your toes and allow your feet to drop naturally out to the sides.

Place your arms at a 45-degree angle away from your body, with your hands relaxed, your palms facing upwards and your fingers slightly curled. Close your eyes. Your entire body should be completely relaxed.

Focus on abdominal breathing, following the rise and fall of your abdomen with each inhalation and exhalation. Allow your breath to move quietly through your nose.

1 **Inhale and lift** your right leg 5cm (2in) off the floor. Hold your breath and focus on your muscles as you hold them up. Exhale, drop your leg to the floor. Take a slow breath and feel the deep relaxation in your leg. Repeat with your left leg.

2 **Inhale and lift** both arms 5cm (2in) off the floor with clenched fists. Hold for a moment. Exhale, drop your arms to the floor. Inhale, and lift your arms with open palms and fingers apart. Hold for a moment. Exhale, lower your arms and relax.

Allow your feet to fall outwards.

"The deeper your relaxation, the more your prana will be restored."

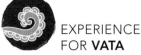

EXPERIENCE FOR **VATA**

Protected during the asanas by the short periods of relaxation, the final relaxation will calm the delicate vata nerves.

EXPERIENCE FOR **PITTA**

The sharp pitta nature becomes balanced by the natural meditative mood that is created by the final relaxation exercises.

EXPERIENCE FOR **KAPHA**

After final relaxation, those with dominant kapha experience a new feeling of lightness that can be maintained with pranayama.

3 **Inhale, squeeze** your glutes and lift your buttocks slightly off the floor. Hold your breath while they are raised. Then, exhale and lower your buttocks back down to the floor again.

4 **Inhale and lift** your chest. Hold your breath for a few seconds. Exhale, lower your chest and release your upper back down to the floor.

5 **Inhale and pull** your shoulders towards your ears. Hold your breath for a few seconds. Exhale and release your shoulders.

6 **Inhale and squeeze** your face muscles tightly together. Hold your breath for a few seconds, then exhale and release.

7 **Inhale, open your** mouth, stick out your tongue, and look up. Hold your breath for a few seconds, exhale, and release.

8 **Inhale and gently** roll your head to one side. Exhale, and turn it to the other side. Repeat several times. Keep your head on the floor and your chin tucked slightly into your throat to allow your neck to relax more.

Breathe slowly and gently in your abdomen.

Relax your palms and fingers.

NOW MOVE ON TO **RELAXATION USING AUTOSUGGESTION**

RELAXATION USING AUTOSUGGESTION

Autosuggestion is the process of the physical body adopting an idea projected by the mind – in this case the act of relaxing. Continue to lie in corpse pose (see pp.160–61) while you perform these exercises; they are the final part of the session.

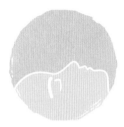

Physical relaxation

🕑 **DURATION:** 7–10 minutes

Take a few slow, rhythmic breaths using your abdomen. Follow this exercise with autosuggestion for 7–10 minutes.

1 **Have a clear mental picture** of your feet, think about the downward pull of gravity. Send a mental command to your feet: *"I am relaxing my feet, I am relaxing my feet, my feet are relaxed."*

2 **Move up your body**, each time visualizing the area you are focusing on, thinking about the pull of gravity and your rhythmic breathing, and sending a command to relax. Start with your ankles, then move all the way up to your scalp.

3 **Finally, relax your internal organs**. Visualize the area, breathe slowly, and send the command to relax to one organ at a time. Start with your abdominal organs, then move up to your brain. Your subconscious conveys the command.

Mental relaxation

🕑 **DURATION:** 1–2 minutes

Mental tension caused by unnecessary worry uses more energy than physical tension. Use this process to release it.

1 **During mental relaxation, breathe slowly** and rhythmically for 1–2 minutes and concentrate on your breathing.

2 **Slowly, your mind will become calm** and you will feel a kind of floating sensation, as if you are as light as a feather – you will feel peace and joy.

AUTOSUGGESTION AND **THE MIND**

Autosuggestion is important as it boosts the mental benefits of the yoga session. Performing pranayama and asanas with short periods of relaxation between works out hyperactivity (rajas, see pp.166–67) or lethargy (tamas), and increases harmony (sattva) in the mind. This effect is augmented by the practice of autosuggestion, and so the mind remains balanced for longer. The practice of raja yoga (covered in the next chapter) will further deepen the benefits of autosuggestion.

Spiritual relaxation

🕒 **DURATION:** 4–5 minutes

The only way to remove all tension and worry is to achieve spiritual relaxation. This process is explained below.

1 **Imagine a quiet**, **crystal-clear lake** and visualize the movements of your thoughts and senses as ripples on the surface of the water.

2 **Gradually let these thought waves** subside so that all that remains is the deep abiding peace of the innermost Self, like seeing through the calm, clear water to the bottom of the lake.

Finishing relaxation

🕒 **DURATION:** 1–2 minutes

The final element of relaxation is the mantra, creating vibratory harmony in the body and mind.

1 **After a few minutes** of spiritual relaxation, the mind will naturally start to move again. Take a few deep breaths and start moving your arms and legs.

2 **Then, stretch out your arms** behind your head. Slowly sit up into a cross-legged position and finish the session by chanting the universal "OM" sound three times. This will help you to maintain physical, mental, and spiritual relaxation for the rest of the day.

"Very little energy is consumed during relaxation. Thus a tremendous amount of energy is being stored and conserved."

SWAMI VISHNUDEVANANDA

POSITIVE
THINKING AND
MEDITATION

"The mind verily is restless, turbulent, strong and unyielding, O Krishna. I deem it as difficult to control as the wind."

BHAGAVAD GITA

AYURVEDA AND **THE MIND**

This chapter covers raja yoga, which uses postive thinking and meditation to help us calm our minds and focus on achieving a state of balance and peace. The three gunas provide insight into the functioning of our minds.

The three gunas

According to the Ayurvedic and yogic scriptures, the mind is a subtle energy field, and is continuously reacting to the information we receive from the physical senses. The three gunas – sattva, rajas, and tamas – are the three energies of the mind. They can be balanced using pranayama and asanas, and that balance can be deepened using mental exercises.

Keeping the mind healthy

As we condition our physical bodies through diet and exercise, our minds are conditioned by the information we receive, whether from friends, family, teachers, or culture, as well as through the type of food we eat (see 'Sattvic diet', pp.64–65). The nature of the mind is inherently sattvic – clear and harmonious. However, by experiencing negative thoughts and emotions, such as greed and fear, or eating an unhealthy diet, the mind loses its pure quality and becomes rajasic (restless and agitated) or tamasic (lethargic and resistant).

A person's mental health depends on how much sattva has been developed in his or her mind. The predominance of rajas and tamas often leads to psychological problems. The goal of both yoga and Ayurveda is to make sattva the predominant guna in the mind. Positive thinking and meditation, both covered in this chapter, remove rajas and tamas, and increase sattva, calming and uplifting the mind.

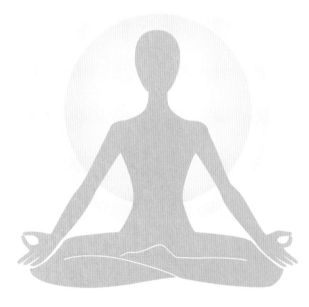

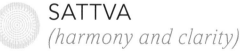 SATTVA
(harmony and clarity)

This is the energy of harmony and clarity. It brings stability, contentment, and peace, as well as revealing truth, making us feel centred and strong. Sattva is dominant in a healthy mind. Under the influence of sattva, a person might be:

- adaptable
- eloquent
- enthusiastic
- positive
- courageous
- independent
- intelligent
- sympathetic
- calm
- contented
- devoted
- humble

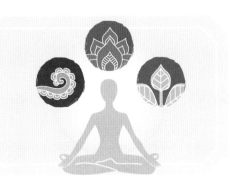

THE **GUNAS** AND THE **DOSHAS**

Regardless of the dominant dosha(s) in a person's constitution, he or she should always be attempting to increase sattva to keep the mind healthy. However, the doshas and gunas combine to affect personality. For example, a person with vata in their constitution may be enthusiastic when sattvic, anxious when rajasic, or depressed when tamasic.

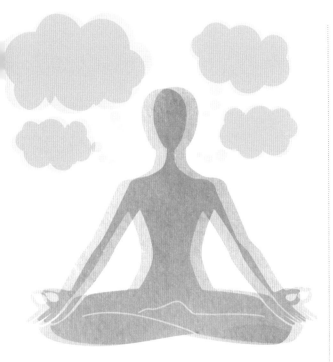

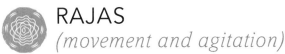

RAJAS
(movement and agitation)

This is the energy of movement, agitation, expansion, and passion. It is needed to bring change, but can delude us into thinking happiness is provided by external pleasures. Excess rajas causes hyperactivity, causing tension and fatigue. Under the influence of rajas, a person might be:

- anxious
- indecisive
- restless
- unreliable
- aggressive
- judgemental
- manipulative
- vain
- compulsive
- dependent
- jealous
- materialistic

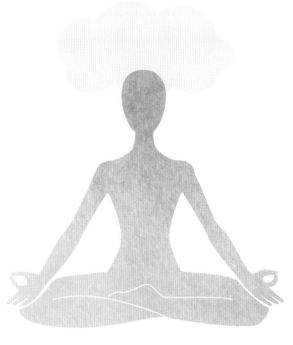

TAMAS
(inertia and contradiction)

This is the energy of inertia, contradiction, and darkness. It is the power of ignorance that makes us resist positive change and creates indifference to our own and other people's wellbeing. In excess it causes lethargy. Under the influence of tamas, a person might be:

- depressed
- dishonest
- prone to addiction
- submissive
- destructive
- dull
- hateful
- judgemental
- apathetic
- lethargic

MONITORING **THE MIND**

The mind is a subtle body influenced by the three gunas, and, like the physical body, must be cared for. This exercise helps you to monitor the state of your mind, and become more aware of the nature of the thoughts that enter it.

Staying motivated

At times, it is difficult to motivate ourselves to perform the daily practices that improve our health. Often this lack of motivation is caused by subconscious beliefs, placed in our minds by the information and conditioning we have received over our lifetimes. However, the knowledge of such beliefs, or even of our minds' conditioning, is not enough to overcome these blockages. We must deeply and courageously look directly into our minds.

Deep introspection

This act of introspection is part of raja yoga. The first step is to develop an awareness that we are indeed conditioned, which we may only vaguely realize. Part of this conditioning may come from a distant past (even past lives, according to Ayurvedic and yogic philosophy), while the rest comes from the people who educated us, from our families and friends, and from the culture we were born into.

We must also become aware of out mental state – the predominance of rajas (agitation) and tamas (resistance). The more we engage in this work, the more we realize how important this awareness is, as our minds affect our physical bodies too – the cells in the body are constantly under the influence of the thoughts in the mind.

DEVELOP AN AWARENESS OF YOUR MENTAL STATE

Sit comfortably in a quiet place with your eyes closed and your back straight. Take a few deep breaths, then begin.

1 **Relax** your mind. Concentrate on the present by focusing on your body and your breath.

2 **Shift** your mental focus within by visualizing an open space or a lake without waves.

3 **Try to observe** your mind, becoming aware of the quality and nature of your thoughts and emotions.

4 **If you see** any negative or disturbing thoughts, do not try to drive them out. Focus on your breathing.

5 **Visualize yourself exhaling** all of the negative thoughts in your mind.

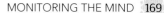

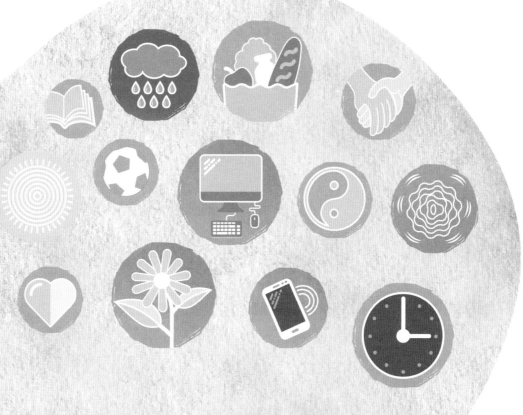

"Be the witness of your thoughts. You will enjoy lasting peace."

SWAMI SIVANANDA

Observe the nature *of the thoughts that enter your mind. Consider whether they are sattvic (harmonious), tamasic, or rajasic.*

NOW MOVE TO
THE MIND AND THE SELF

THE MIND AND **THE SELF**

Ayurveda teaches us that we are not our minds, but rather a separate consciousness, also called the Self. This exercise will help you to start to realize the separation between the mind and consciousness.

What is the Self?

Both yoga and Ayurveda teach that the root cause of disease is the failure to understand our true nature. We might think that we are a physical body with a mind – a personality – but this is not the case. We are consciousness – "the Self" – a silent witness that uses the mind to express itself in the world of forms.

Only once you realize that you are not your mind (in the same way that you are not your physical body) can you stop identifying with your mind's moods and habits. The ultimate purpose of yoga and Ayurveda is not to control the mind, which is fighting a lost battle, but to dissolve its thoughts and content, so that we experience our true nature – pure consciousness – a state of ultimate bliss.

Knowing the theory behind the separation of the mind and the Self is easy, but a true realization takes a long time to achieve.

> *"When you meditate, some irrelevant thoughts may enter your mind. Ignore them. They will pass away."*
>
> SWAMI SIVANANDA

SEPARATION FROM THE MIND

This exercise will help you come to terms with the idea that you are separate from your mind. Make sure you are sitting in a comfortable position in a quiet place. Take a few deep breaths, then begin.

1 **Scan your body** for tensions while you breathe rhythmically.

2 **Create space within** yourself by visualizing a space between your body and your thoughts.

3 **Watch your thoughts** come and go in a never-ending motion. The mind is like a monkey, jumping from one thought to another in an uncontrolled way. See how compulsive the movement of thoughts is. Become an unaffected witness, observing your mind.

4 **Realize that the part** of you that is observing the thoughts is different to the thoughts themselves.

5 **Repeat mentally,** "I witness my thoughts, and therefore I am not my thoughts."

6 **Feel the calmness** and expansion that come with this realization.

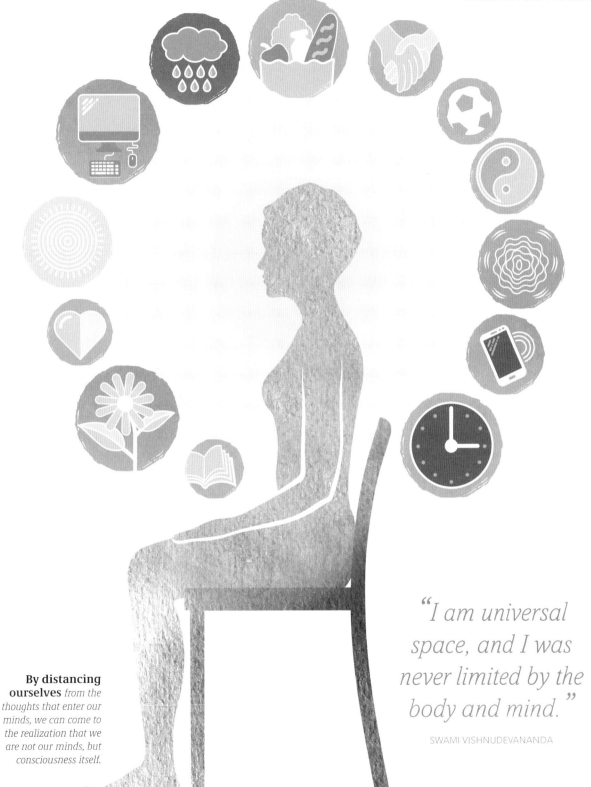

By distancing ourselves *from the thoughts that enter our minds, we can come to the realization that we are not our minds, but consciousness itself.*

"I am universal space, and I was never limited by the body and mind."

SWAMI VISHNUDEVANANDA

POSITIVE THINKING

Now that we have a picture of how the mind functions, we can examine the practices that pacify, balance, and uplift it by increasing sattva. The first of these is to dwell in positivity by having positive sensory experiences and positive thoughts.

Positive sensory experiences

Positive experiences leave a good impression in our minds, increasing our levels of sattva (harmony). Below are some examples of ways you can have positive sensory experiences. Try to do these practices as often as you can – maybe once a week or more.

- **Go on a woodland or countryside walk** by yourself. Connect to the five elements, such as the dense earth or the warm sun. Become aware of the infinite space all around you, and allow your mind to expand into its immensity.
- **Examine a beautiful work of art** that you are particularly drawn to in a gallery. Let your eyes feast on the richness of the colours, the power of the lines.
- **Listen to spiritual music,** such as mantra chanting recordings. Feel how this music has the power to pull your mind inside, and put you in touch with the highest of all sounds, the silence of the soul.

We can also reduce the amount of rajasic and tamasic impressions we receive from the media by limiting our time on our phones or computers, or at least be selective about what we choose to watch or listen to.

"Thought is a dynamic force; it shapes your destiny. Entertain pure and noble thoughts always."

SWAMI SIVANANDA

Positive thoughts

The second form of dwelling in positivity is through positive thinking. This exercise requires you to focus on improving the quality of your inner world, independent of outer circumstances.

This is important, as dwelling on external desires keeps us in a state of wanting, which leads to a sense of emptiness and frustration. Only through building a positive inner world can we find lasting contentment.

HOW TO USE POSITIVE AFFIRMATIONS

Choose one or two positive affirmations, or use them all. Repeat them three times a day – when you wake, at a convenient time during the day, and before bed. Say them slowly and clearly, with determination, and in a relaxed state of mind, as if talking to a friend. Have no expectation of immediate results.

My will is pure and irresistible.

My mind is clear and calm like a lake without waves.

My heart is filled with gratitude towards life.

All is happening for my good, to make me strong and aware.

My heart is filled with compassion towards all beings.

I accept myself as I am.

I open myself to the light of my Higher Self.

I surrender to the Self within.

I am not the doer. I am an instrument in the hands of the divine.

I open myself to the guidance of my Higher Self (or God).

REFINING **OUR VALUES**

The practice of positive thinking goes deeper than using affirmations. The path of raja yoga encourages us to uplift our minds through the practice of positive attitudes towards both ourselves and others.

Gaining sattva with our actions

To develop sattva (harmony) we need to work on our character. For this we must follow the principle of dharma, living the right way (see p.8). We need to realize that we are not separate from others, but part of a whole, and whatever we do to others, we do to ourselves. There are ten ethical practices that we can try to follow.

How to practise

Choose one of the practices described here and work with it systematically for one month. For example, you could work on "Do not harm" and do the following:

- **Count how many** times each day you indulged in violence (whether harsh words, anger, or harmful thoughts)
- **Reflect on** what behaviour you could replace it with
- **Think of** a person that is an example of non-violence
- **Make the** decision for yourself: I choose to always be peaceful
- **Reflect on** the benefits of peaceful behaviour.

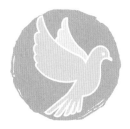

1 DO NOT HARM

This means seeking to do good for others, wishing them well, and avoiding causing harm through thoughts, words, and actions. Swami Sivananda said, "Wish good to all beings, this purifies the mind."

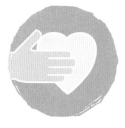

2 BE TRUTHFUL

Being truthful to ourselves is essential, as without this we are incapable of deep introspection. Being truthful to others is also essential, since respecting our values is the foundation of a healthy mind.

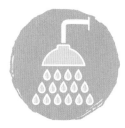

6 MAINTAIN CLEANLINESS

A clean body is achieved through asanas, diet (ideally vegetarian), and daily hygiene (see pp.34–35). Keeping the mind clean involves avoiding tamasic impressions, and not indulging in gossip, criticism, or negative thinking.

7 BE CONTENTED

Contentment is being grateful for what life has given us, and showing a willingness to work with it. It requires an attitude of patience, knowing that change is slow, and the fruits of practice take a long time to show.

"Think deeply, decide correctly, act carefully,
speak truthfully, behave properly.
You will be peaceful and successful."

SWAMI SIVANANDA

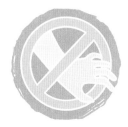

3 DON'T STEAL

Taking what belongs to others makes the mind tamasic (resistant). This includes intellectual property and material possessions, as well as being careful not to take too much from the world without giving back.

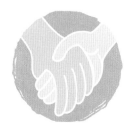

4 BE SEXUALLY MODERATE

Ayurveda and yoga teach moderation in sexuality, so that sexual energy can build up and be transformed into mental strength. Full practice (the diversion of all sexual energy) is only possible with systematic yoga practice.

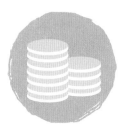

5 LIVE MODESTLY

Greed for material wealth prevents us from connecting to the Self, while the clutter created by having many possessions makes it harder to calm the mind. Gratefully accept what you have, and don't take more than you need.

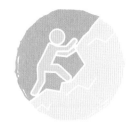

8 BE DISCIPLINED

To reach full mental health in the form of lasting peace and joy is a worthy goal, and so requires many sacrifices. This can only be done with the self-discpline to stay focused on this goal and face the challenges of life.

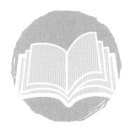

9 STRIVE FOR SELF-IMPROVEMENT

The mind can be nurtured by reading spiritual books, listening to uplifting discourse, and repeating mantras. It is not about accumulating knowledge, but gaining a greater understanding of oneself.

10 SURRENDER TO A HIGHER POWER

Willpower alone is not enough to break the pattern of fear and ignorance – we must accept help by opening ourselves up to a higher influence we can trust. This may be a form of the divine or a spiritual teacher.

MEDITATION PRACTICE

Meditation goes beyond positive thinking. It teaches us that we already have all we need, and that, by creating space and silence within, we can experience the peace and bliss of our true Self.

MENTAL **BENEFITS**

- **Focuses the mind,** so we can see into our inner world.
- **Removes tamas** (resistance).
- **Helps overcome rajas** (agitation).
- **Increases sattva** (harmony).
- **Empties the mind** of thoughts.

How to meditate

Meditation requires focusing your attention on one object. Practise daily for 20–30 minutes. Find a clean, quiet place (a cluttered or dirty environment will distract the mind) and sit in a comfortable position with your back straight, then begin.

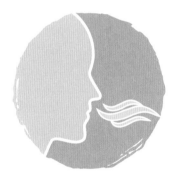

1 **Focus on your breath.** Start with a few deep and slow breaths to trigger a relaxation response in your nervous system.

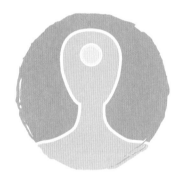

2 **Focus on your third eye** or the centre of your chest (see below) to ground your mind and start channelling its energy.

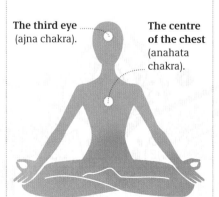

The third eye (ajna chakra).

The centre of the chest (anahata chakra).

3 **Slow your breathing** to a minimum, inhale and exhale silently for 3–4 seconds. Clearly instruct your mind to slow down and relax.

"Do not force the mind to meditate. Understand the mind first; study the three gunas. Only then will meditation be smooth and easy."

SWAMI SIVANANDA

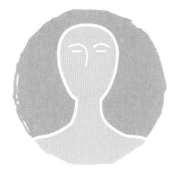

4 **Focus your chosen point** of concentration. This should be one of the following subjects:

An object *that you find uplifting – this might be a shaft of light, an open space, a flower, or even the ocean*

A mantra *that you have chosen – see pp.178–81 for examples of different types of mantras and how to use them*

Your mind *– observe your thoughts without reacting to them, even if they are negative or disturbing.*

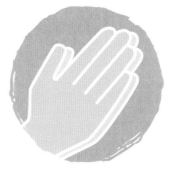

5 **Finish your meditation** session on a feeling of gratefulness and/or a short prayer for the world.

SIGNS OF PROGRESS

Your progress is not necessarily measured by the your success in focusing your mind, or by whether you have special experiences during your meditation practice. You will know that you are on the right track mainly by the way you feel the rest of the day:

- **Your mind** will be generally more calm, positive and balanced
- **Your emotions** will be more steady and of a sattvic nature
- **You will feel** inspired to serve others
- **You will be more** tolerant and compassionate towards others
- **You will adapt** and adjust more easily to change
- **You will develop** a broader perspective of life
- **You will be more** accepting of life and yourself.

THE POWER OF MANTRAS

The challenge of meditation is to maintain your attention as long as you can. The mind has a tendency to get distracted, so a helpful tool to prevent this is a mantra.

What are mantras?

Mantras are to the mind what asanas are to the body – they can reshape and transform it in a positive way. A mantra is a sound or phrase, and the practice of using mantras is simple – just repeat the sound or phrase loudly, quietly, or mentally. These repetitions give the mind energy, while the vibrations created by saying the mantra overpower and dissolve negative thought patterns, replacing them with positive ones.

Repeating mantras requires patience, and a mantra may have to be repeated many thousands of times before its power is released. It is like creating a fire – it needs to constantly be fed with wood so that it burns brighter and brighter.

There are many types of mantras you can chant (see pp.180–81). It is often best to learn the pronunciation from a teacher, so you may want to start with a simple mantra, such as "OM".

MENTAL BENEFITS

- **Cleanses**, soothes, and rejuvenates the mind.
- **Turns the mind** inwards, making it pure and peaceful.
- **Sublimates** selfish emotion, turning it into love.
- **Allows one** to realize the unity of all forms connected to the source of life.

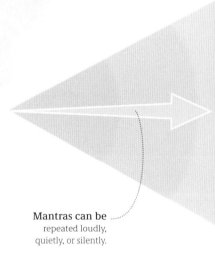

Mantras can be repeated loudly, quietly, or silently.

"This sound, which is held in the field of our consciousness, liberates us."

MANTRA SHASTRA

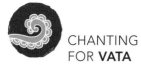

CHANTING FOR **VATA**

Those with a lot of vata in their constitution benefit from a slow repetition of their mantra to calm their hyperactive tendencies.

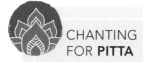

CHANTING FOR **PITTA**

To counteract their sharp natures, those with a lot of pitta in their constitution should repeat their mantra with a feeling of reverence.

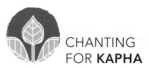

CHANTING FOR **KAPHA**

Repeating their mantra quickly is best for those with dominant kapha. They may start loudly to overcome any sluggishness.

Repeating mantras

Mantra practice should be done daily for 20–30 minutes. Start by sitting in a clean, quiet place in a comfortable position. Ideally, take a shower first and wear clean clothes. See pp.180–81 for information about which mantra to use.

1 RELAX

Close your eyes. Relax your body and mind by focusing on your breathing.

2 FOCUS

Focus on the present, don't think about the past and future.

3 REPEAT

Repeat your mantra silently within.

4 SYNCHRONIZE

Synchronize your mantra repetitions with your breath.

5 MEANING

Focus on the sound, the meaning, or the deity associated with your mantra.

MANTRAS AND **MENTAL HEALTH**

According to Ayurveda, mantras can be an effective way to alleviate mental-health issues. The energy of the mantra breaks down negative thought patterns without requiring analysis of the problems causing them. Speech-based therapies often require talking about problems, which may bring greater awareness of their nature and causes, but may not necessarily give one the power to detach and move on.

NOW MOVE ON TO
CHOOSING A MANTRA

Choosing a mantra

The process of deciding which mantra you want to use is largely intuitive – you may feel attracted to the sound of the mantra, or feel inspired by the deity it represents. You might also choose the one that sounds and feels right when you say it.

The two main types of mantras are nirguna mantras and saguna mantras. Both types should be used in the same way. Pick one mantra and work with it systematically. Repeat it during your meditation session, and use it throughout the day to focus and elevate the mind, and to protect it from the negative energies of rajas (agitation) and tamas (resistance).

> *"Repeat your mantra at all times, even while you study, play, and work, while you eat and rest. The mantra is the source of all inspiration and strength."*
>
> SWAMI SIVANANDA

NIRGUNA MANTRAS

The powerful vibrations generated by these mantras activate the chakras (energy centres of the body, see p.176), tuning them in the same way that you would an instrument. The outcome is an inner awakening, in which we realize our connection to the greater body of the universe.

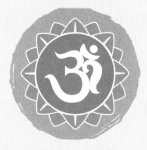

OM
The sound of creation

The OM sound brings inspiration and intuition. Most mantras begin with "OM", but it can also be chanted by itself. Swami Sivananda says the OM is "your spiritual food, ... derive energy from OM, rely on OM, meditate on OM – you will attain the highest knowledge."

SO'HAM
The essence of breath

The sound of this mantra can be synchronized with the breath (inhale on "SO" and exhale on "HAM"). It awakens the power of discrimination, asserting again and again that we are not our outer form, but rather a witness and dweller in our form.

SAGUNA MANTRAS

These mantras connect us to the inner self through the medium of deities. In Hinduism, each deity is a personification of a different power of the universe, for example, Siva represents transformation. Recognizing and connecting to these powers is a great aid to psychological healing.

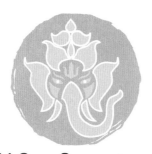

OM Gam Ganapataye Namah

Deity: **Ganesha**
Deity's essence: **Removal of obstacles**

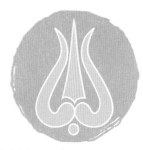

OM Namah Sivaya

Deity: **Siva**
Deity's essence: **Transformation**

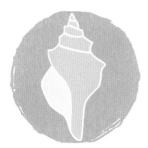

OM Namo Narayanaya

Deity: **Vishnu**
Deity's essence: **Benevolence and peace**

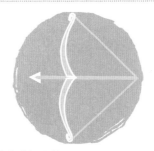

OM Shri Ramaya Namah

Deity: **Rama**
Deity's essence: **Duty and harmony**

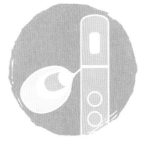

OM Namo Bhagavate Vasudevaya

Deity: **Krishna**
Deity's essence: **Joy and love**

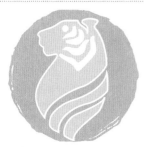

OM Shri Durgayai Namah

Deity: **Durga**
Deity's essence: **Divine protection and righteousness**

OM Shri Mahalakshmyai Namah

Deity: **Lakshmi**
Deity's essence: **Beauty, generosity, and abundance**

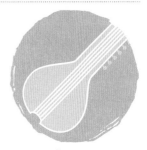

OM Aim Saraswatyai Namah

Deity: **Saraswati**
Deity's essence: **Creation**

KARMA YOGA

Focusing the mind during meditation can be a real challenge. A good way to increase concentration and sattva (harmony) in these circumstances is through karma yoga – the practice of selfless service.

Balancing the mind through selfless service

Karma yoga requires a person to act in the service of others without expectation of material gain, acknowledgment, or fame. The action must be performed for its own sake.

The change of focus from oneself to others diverts the mind from self-centred thought patterns. What's more, the process actually serves to balance the mind, because we are freed from the biggest source of psychological problems – the ego, which creates a sense of separation from others. When we open ourselves up to the pain of other beings (humans, animals, or even the planet as a whole), we can relate to them with compassion and empathy. This uplifts our minds and opens our hearts. After all, the purpose of human life goes beyond individual wellbeing – it aims at the expression of a higher consciousness through the individual. Our dharma (duty to live the right way) is thus to serve and work for the good of all beings. This will give us lasting peace and a sense of purpose in life.

How to practise karma yoga
Think how you can best use your energy, time, material resources, or knowledge for the good of society. This will cleanse your mind and bring you peace. When helping others, try to do the things shown around the image on the right.

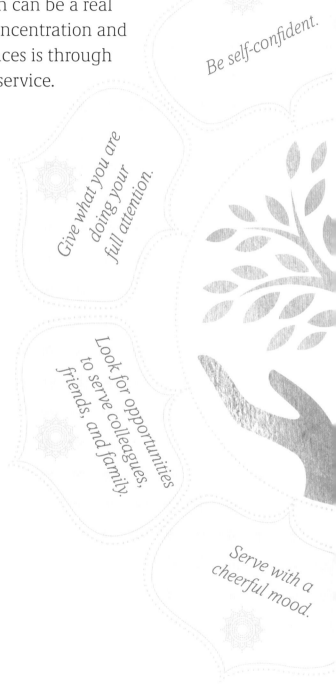

Be self-confident.

Give what you are doing your full attention.

Look for opportunities to serve colleagues, friends, and family.

Serve with a cheerful mood.

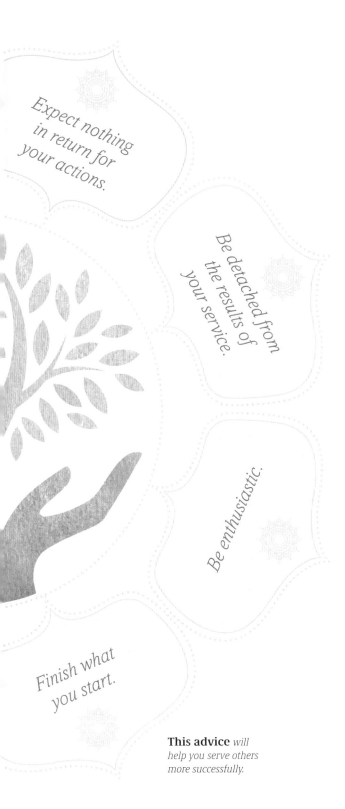

Expect nothing in return for your actions.

Be detached from the results of your service.

Be enthusiastic.

Finish what you start.

This advice *will help you serve others more successfully.*

"*Life is meant for service and not for self-seeking. Hold your life for the service of others. The more energy you expend in elevating others, the more universal energy will flow into you.* "

SWAMI SIVANANDA

EXAMPLES OF SERVICE

Swami Sivananda recommended practising karma yoga for a few hours each week. Some examples of selfless service are:

• **Helping in a spiritual** or charitable institution once a week

• **Visiting elderly people** in an old people's home and lifting them up with positive words or spiritual readings

• **Saying encouraging** and compassionate words to friends in distress

• **Thinking how** you can best use your energy, education, or wealth to improve society, and then acting on it.

THE **BIGGER PICTURE**

Ayurveda and yoga follow the philosophy of unity, asserting that all beings are essentially one, even though they appear as separate forms. This understanding gives us the strength to deal with life's challenges.

The path to moksha

We have been introduced to the idea that the consciousness resides in the Self (see pp.170–171). Yoga and Ayurveda teach that this consciousness is connected to the consciousness of all beings.

The realization of this truth is called moksha (see p.9), and it allows us to experience the bliss of our true being. It is not easy to break the illusion that all beings are separate. Even if it may seem like a distant goal, we benefit from regularly contemplating this truth.

Positivity during pain

We can learn from pain and discomfort, as these remind us of the transience of our physical forms. While good health is a blessing, it may keep us attached to our bodies and minds. The poor health of the body can act as a catalyst for moksha, making us aware of the Self beyond the form of the body and mind. This creates positivity in periods of poor physical health – we can use this time as an opportunity for spiritual growth.

Beyond physical existence

Once we realize that we are spiritual beings having a physical experience, the way we relate to death changes. The fear of ceasing to exist is deep-set within us, but knowing we exist beyond our physical and mental forms helps us face this fear with greater ease. According to yoga, death is the separation of the Self from the physical body. It is an experience like dreaming, where the physical form is lost, but the consciousness continues to exist.

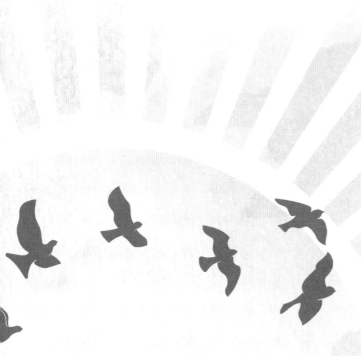

POSITIVE AFFIRMATIONS
FOR SPIRITUAL HEALTH

Repeat these affirmations during your meditation, or any time during the day when you want to centre yourself and feel peace:

- **I am the Self,** which is independent of the body and mind.
- **I am the pure light** of consciousness.
- **I am free.**
- **I was never born,** I will never die.
- **I am bliss** absolute.

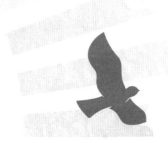

"See life as a whole. All life is one. The world is one home and we are all members of one human family. All creation is an organic whole. No one is independent from that whole."

SWAMI SIVANANDA

SEEING AN
AYURVEDIC
PRACTITIONER

"A physician must use their knowledge as a light to enter into the heart of a person."

CHARAKA

AYURVEDIC **DIAGNOSIS**

Seeing an Ayurvedic practitioner can help you if you want to learn more about your constitution, optimize your health, or get treatment if you are unwell.

Holistic assessment

An Ayurvedic practitioner looks at the whole picture of your health during an assessment, and tries to achieve a full understanding of you as a person. To do this, he or she will determine your constitution, appraise the balance of your doshas, the health of your dhatus (tissues), the strength of your agni (digestive fire) as well as your ojas (immunity), and sattva (mental harmony). This will involve asking questions on topics such as your lifestyle, diet, personal and professional life, as well as your medical history, and any current problems. Knowing your constitution will provide insight into which doshas are most likely to be increased and which therapies will suit you best, while your level of ojas and state of mind influence your ability to recover well.

Preventing illness

In Ayurveda, disease is considered to be a symptom of an imbalance in the body – an elevated dosha, weak agni, or the presence of ama (toxins) can affect your tissues and eventually cause illness. Ayurveda aims to restore balance in the early stages before disease can manifest. This means treating unspecific symptoms such as general feelings of unease or discomfort.

Your constitution is assessed to determine the proportions of vata, pitta, and kapha in your body and mind.

Dosha imbalances in your body are diagnosed and their extent is determined.

Your agni (digestive fire) is vital for many bodily processes. Healthy agni leads to healthy dhatus.

Dhatus (tissues) are examined for specific problems during a physical examination (see p.190–91). Healthy dhatus indicate resilience to disease.

Your ojas (immunity) determines how much protection your dhatus have from disease, and helps support prana (vital energy).

Your mind's state is determined by its levels of sattva (see pp.166–67). This affects your immunity to, and recovery from, disease.

Your lifestyle – when and how often you eat, sleep, exercise, etc. – affects the function of your body.

Your diet – what and how much you eat – is assessed to determine how it impacts your doshas and agni.

Your personal and professional situation has a large impact on the health of your body and mind.

Your age affects how resilient you are and which doshas are most likely to be irritated or elevated.

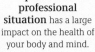

Your physical strength is an indication of your dhatus' resilience to disease.

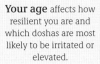

Your elimination of malas (sweat, urine, and stools) indicates how well your body is functioning.

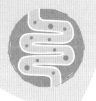

To diagnose your state of health, *it is important for an Ayurvedic practitioner to assess these aspects of your life, mind, and body.*

Treating and rebalancing

The Ayurvedic practitioner's aim is to both treat immediate health issues and help you to stay well afterwards. After assessing your symptoms and diagnosing which doshas and tissues are involved, he or she will recommend dietary and lifestyle changes to treat the root cause of the problem. The practitioner may also treat you with body treatments, nourishing or cleansing therapies, or Ayurvedic herbal medicines. The goal of this comprehensive regimen is to help prevent the same imbalances returning.

> *"The causes of disease are placed into three groups: unsuitable use of the senses, faulty judgement, and the effects of time."*
>
> SWAMI SIVANANDA

NOW MOVE ON TO
YOUR EXAMINATION

YOUR **EXAMINATION**

After asking questions, the practitioner will do a physical examination. They will take your pulse and examine your body to assess you constitution, look for signs of dosha imbalances, and to determine the state of your dhatus (tissues).

Checking your pulse

Your pulse is one of the primary indicators of the state of your doshas. The practitioner uses three fingers to find your pulse, and its location will provide information about your doshas.

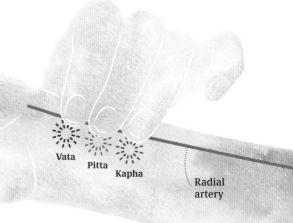

Vata   Pitta   Kapha

Radial artery

1 **The practitioner** places three fingers over your radial artery. In women, the pulse of the left wrist is taken first; in men, the right.

2 **He or she presses** down firmly until they cannot feel your pulse, then they release their fingers slowly and note which finger first feels your pulse return.

3 **A strong pulse** under the forefinger indicates strong vata; the middle finger indicates strong pitta; and the ring finger strong kapha.

PULSE PATTERN

The nature of your pulse (see right) can help to identify which dosha(s) are dominant in your constitution.

A vata pulse is quick and changes speed, like a winding snake.

A pitta pulse is strong, like the movement of a jumping frog.

A kapha pulse feels full, like the stately movement of a swan.

Examining the body

The tongue, eyes, nails, and skin are some of the most common parts of the body for a practitioner to examine because they can show early signs of dosha imbalance, weak agni (digestive fire), or ama (toxins). The practitioner may also examine your chest and abdomen.

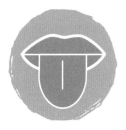

TONGUE

If your tongue is dry, you may have a vata imbalance. If it is deep red or yellowish in colour, it could signal a pitta imbalance, while a white coating indicates kapha imbalance. A thick coating may indicate ama.

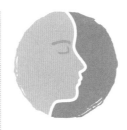

SKIN

If your skin is dry, cracked, and rough, you may have a vata imbalance. Red, hot, or sensitive skin with rashes can indicate pitta imbalance, while pale, cool, or clammy skin can indicate a kapha imbalance.

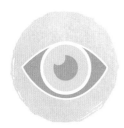

EYES

Your eyes may be restless, indicating vata imbalance; yellowish and sensitive to light, indicating pitta imbalance; or watering and dull, indicating an imbalance of kapha.

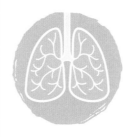

CHEST

Your chest could be examined to check for abnormal sounds, such as wheezing. The presence of large amounts of mucous can indicate excess kapha.

NAILS

Your nails will be strong and healthy if agni is healthy, but longitudinal lines can indicate your body is not absorbing food effectively.

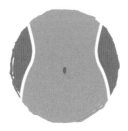

ABDOMEN

Your abdomen or any tender part of your body may be palpated to assess damage or injury. This can help the practitioner determine the state of your tissues.

"Ayurveda is the science of life. It shows the way to remove diseases, to maintain sound health, and to attain longevity."

SWAMI SIVANANDA

BODY **TREATMENTS**

These treatments aim to pacify the doshas and strengthen the dhatus (tissues). They require the application of therapeutic substances – such as oils or powders – directly onto the body.

Healing and soothing

The direct application of therapeutic substances onto the body helps rejuvenate the dhatus (tissues) and supports the function of the entire body or the specific part of the body that is treated. Body treatments can also be used to soothe irritated doshas (cases of minor dosha imbalance). To do this, a practitioner will choose a therapeutic substance that pacifies the relevant dosha – such as giving someone with irritated vata a massage using sesame oil.

IMPORTANT NOTE

These treatments should not be done on a full stomach or immediately after eating.

If you are pregnant, seek the advice of an Ayurvedic practitioner before having any treatments, as some may not be suitable.

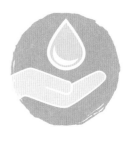

CLASSIC OIL MASSAGE

Known as "abhyanga" in Sanskrit, this can be a full-body massage or a partial massage of the head and face, back, or feet. Warm herbal oil is used according to the season and the constitution of the person treated. Oil massages are particularly beneficial for vata as they moisturize and calm the nervous system, strengthen the dhatus, alleviate pain, reduce joint stiffness, boost immunity, and balance hormones. They are not advised in cases of fever or ama.

STEAM BATH

This is a classic therapy that uses wet heat. It aids the digestion of the oil and herbs applied during a massage, helping to eliminate sweat and pacify vata and kapha. In cases of strongly elevated kapha, dry heat may be more appropriate (see pp.194–95). All massages should ideally be followed by a steam bath, but steam baths can also be performed separately.

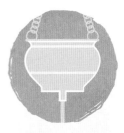

OIL POURING ON THE FOREHEAD

Known as "shirodhara" in Sanskrit, this is a treatment in which warm oil (for all three doshas) or buttermilk (to cool down pitta) is poured onto the forehead in a continuous stream. It has a powerful effect on the mind, providing deep relaxation, improved concentration and sleep, and easing headaches and depression. It is best done three times in a single session by an experienced therapist as part of a full therapeutic regimen, such as panchakarma (see pp.194–95).

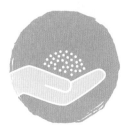

DRY POWDER
MASSAGE

This massage treatment uses a powder made from kapha-reducing herbs, such as basil and sage, mixed with chickpea flour and salt. This alleviates problems associated with elevated kapha (such as excess fat tissue or a slow metabolism) due to its drying, heating, and stimulating qualities. Dry powder massages are a good alternative to oil massages if you have ama, but they should not be done on areas of the body affected by skin irritations or rashes.

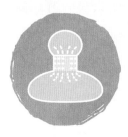

HERBAL BOLUS
MASSAGE

A muslin bag (or bolus) filled with herbal preparations and heated in oil is used to massage the body – the heat aids the absorption of the active ingredients in the herbs. To pacify vata, herbs, oil, milk, and rice are combined in order to provide a nourishing effect; for pitta, a mixture of herbs and pitta oil are used for a cooling effect; and for kapha, the bolus is filled with herbs and oil that provide a heating, stimulating effect.

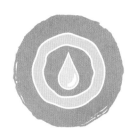

LOCAL OIL
TREATMENT

In this treatment, a ring made from chickpea flour and water is laid on a specific joint or area of the body and slowly filled with heated herbal oil. A therapist gently stirs the oil as it is poured. The oil is replaced when it starts to cool. Local oil treatment is used for treating slipped or worn discs, lumbago, joint or nerve pain, menstrual pain, and arthritis. It can also be performed on the chest over the heart as a therapy for high blood pressure.

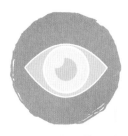

EYE
BATH

As with the local oil treatment (see left), eye baths require a ring made from chickpea flour and water, but this time it is placed over the eyes. The therapist pours lukewarm ghee into the ring and the patient is then asked to open his or her eyes and move them around. Eye baths are used to help soothe irritated eyes, help preserve healthy eyesight, and treat certain eye diseases. Do not have an eye bath if you have been diagnosed with glaucoma.

THERAPEUTIC ACTIONS

Ayurvedic treatments are designed to perform one or more of the six therapeutic actions described in the classical texts (see below). Your practitioner will select an appropriate body treatment for you based on the desired action. For example, if you have excess kapha in the form of being overweight, reducing and drying therapies, such as fasting and dry powder massage, will suit your needs best. The six actions are as follows:

- **Reducing** therapies remove excess tissue and increase lightness
- **Nourishing** therapies, such as massage with nourishing oils, build up tissue and increase heaviness, oiliness, and cold
- **Drying** therapies counteract excess oil, water, and stickiness, and have a reducing effect
- **Oiling** therapies have a lubricating action that softens and moisturizes the body
- **Fomentation** therapies induce sweating to help counteract stiffness, heaviness, and cold
- **Blocking** therapies reduce the flow of liquids (eg. in diarrhoea or menorrhagia). They increase cold, slowness, dryness, fineness, and stability.

PANCHAKARMA

Meaning "five actions" in Sanskrit, panchakarma is a set of five cleansing, detoxifying treatments that remove elevated doshas and rejuvenate the whole body.

Purifying therapies

Panchakarma restores energy, cleanses the tissues, and reinstates the natural balance of the doshas. While body treatments can soothe irritated doshas, panchakarma treatments actively remove elevated doshas (doshas that have become seriously unbalanced and can affect the tissues over time). The effects of panchakarma can be felt for a year or longer if the proper diet and lifestyle advice is followed. Ideally, panchakarma treatments should be performed at the change of each season to get rid of the doshas. Nowadays, it is generally recommended to have panchakarma treatments once a year in spring or autumn.

Types of panchakarma

There are five therapies in classical panchakarma (see right); these can be intense, and require good health. In modern times, Kerala panchakarma is more commonly used – it is less taxing, and can even be prescribed to the elderly or unwell. Most Ayurvedic treatment centres offer Kerala panchakarma.

A full panchakarma treatment should be performed by an experienced Ayurvedic practitioner in an inpatient environment.

CLASSICAL PANCHAKARMA

VAMANA (EMESIS) — 1

Medical emesis, or "vamana" in Sanskrit, eliminates elevated kapha and pitta from the respiratory and gastrointestinal tract. It involves giving medicines to induce therapeutic vomiting.

VIRECHANA (PURGATION) — 2

Medical purgation, or "virechana" in Sanskrit, eliminates elevated pitta from the small intestine. It involves evacuating the bowels by giving the patient a herbal purgative or laxative.

BASTI (ENEMA) — 3

Herbal enemas, or "basti" in Sanskrit, are mostly used to eliminate elevated vata, but can be used to reduce pitta or kapha. Oil-based enemas have a nourishing effect, while water-based enemas are cleansing.

NASYA (OILING NOSTRILS) — 4

Nasal passage lubrication, or "nasya" in Sanskrit, eliminates elevated kapha and reduces vata and pitta. The treatment is administered by pouring herbal oil into the sinuses through the nostrils.

RAKTA MOKSHA (BLEEDING) — 5

Blood letting, or "rakta moksha" in Sanskrit, eliminates blood as a tissue and removes elevated pitta. In modern times, it is best done by donating blood or leech therapy.

KERALA
PANCHAKARMA

1 ABHYANGA (OIL MASSAGE)

Oil massages (see p.192) are preparatory treatments for Kerala panchakarma. They are effective at soothing vata, and can also be used to soothe pitta and kapha if the correct oils are used.

2 INNER OILING

This process requires the ingestion of ghee, and only rarely oil. It is used as a preparatory treatment, lubricating the body for purgation and enema treatments.

3 VIRECHANA (PURGATION)

Medical purgation treatments are often included in Kerala panchakarma. They eliminate elevated pitta from the small intestine. Inner and outer oiling must be used as preparation.

4 BASTI (ENEMA)

An enema treatment with oil, herbal oil, or herbal decoction is often included in Kerala panchakarma as well as in classical panchakarma. It eliminates elevated vata.

5 OTHER BODY TREATMENTS

Body treatments, such as oil pouring onto the forehead, or herbal bolus or dry powder massage (see pp.192–193), may be included to help to soothe irritated doshas.

PREPARING FOR **PANCHAKARMA**

Ama (toxins) should be treated (i.e. digested) before undergoing either form of panchakarma. Classical panchakarma requires proper preparation with oil massages and inner oiling, mostly using herbal or pure ghee. Oil massages and inner oiling are included in the main part of Kerala panchakarma.

Vata can be irritated by treatments from both forms of panchakarma, so great care is taken to soothe it. Travel, change of time zone, and climate are all vata-irritating factors, so if you are travelling for your treatment (eg. Westerners going to India) allow ample time to acclimatize beforehand.

After panchakarma, give yourself time to recover before you resume your daily life. Don't plan any holidays or intense work for the following 2–3 weeks.

AYURVEDIC **MEDICINES**

In Ayurveda, all substances have a therapeutic effect and can be used as medicine. This includes herbs and foods when given in medicinal doses.

Healing effects

Ayurveda has a vast knowledge of India's indigenous herbs, and treatment with these herbs is a mainstay. Herbs and other therapeutic substances are selected by an Ayurvedic practitioner according to six criteria that determine the effects it has on you (see right). These effects include pacifying doshas, healing dhatus (tissues), strengthening agni (digestive fire), and influencing the mind and body in general.

Forms of herbal preparation

There are many types of herbal preparations used in Ayurveda. The most common of these are listed below.

- **Powdered herbs** are best taken with hot water (for all doshas), warm milk (for vata), ghee (for pitta), or honey (for kapha).
- **Herbal pills or capsules** can be taken in the same way as powdered herbs (see above).
- **Decoctions** are water-based extracts of the herb's active ingredients. They can be taken orally with salt, honey, or sugar. Herbs are added to ghee or oils by making a decoction first.
- **Herbal wines**, known as asavas or arishtas, are fermented infusions or decoctions. They aid digestion and absorption of the herbs even if agni is weak.
- **Herbal oils** are applied to the body topically via massage. Ayurvedic oils are rich in healing herbs: up to 5kg (10lb) of herbs are processed into 1 litre (1¾ pints) of oil, ensuring that your body receives a large quantity of healing herbs, even from a single massage.

TASTE

The effect a substance has on you starts with its taste. Each taste has various therapeutic actions. For example, the sweet taste builds tissue; sour is slightly purgative; salty promotes digestion; pungent is cleansing and stimulates agni; bitter helps lower fever; astringent promotes wound healing.

QUALITIES

Ayurvedic medicine refers to 20 main qualities in pairs of opposites, such as light–heavy and dull–sharp. These qualities are used to create an effect or counteract an unwanted property. For example, too much dryness in the body can be counteracted with ghee, which has the "oily" quality.

POTENCY

Potency refers to whether a substance has a heating effect or cooling effect. A substance's potency is important because it is not changed by digestion. Hot potency pacifies vata and kapha and elevates pitta, while cold potency pacifies pitta and elevates vata and kapha.

POST-DIGESTIVE TASTE

We are unable to perceive this taste, which develops after the digestive process. The six tastes are consolidated into just three: sweet, sour, and pungent. Post-digestive tastes have a more significant, longer-lasting effect than pre-digestive tastes.

ACTIONS ON THE BODY

Each substance can have its own specific effects on the body's functions, such as reducing fever, cough, or weakness, building or reducing tissue, stopping flow, or removing blockages. It may also have a reducing or elevating effect on a particular dosha – for example, sugar has an elevating effect on kapha dosha.

SPECIAL PROPERTIES

Some substances have special properties that cannot be explained by its other aspects (taste, quality, etc.). For example, ghee has the special property of stimulating agni despite being cooling and heavy (and thus in theory being likely to weaken agni).

RESTORATIVE MEDICINES

Ayurveda includes a branch of therapy called "rasayana" (or "rejuvenation") which focuses on restoring tissue health and generating resilient tissue in the long term. Healthy tissues and organs are the body's best defense against disease, as disease cannot manifest itself in healthy tissues, even if the doshas are irritated or elevated.

Rasayana is the last step in Ayurvedic treatment. These medicines are given after agni has been strengthened, ama (toxins) has been removed, and the doshas balanced (for example, after panchakarma). This ensures that the body is able to fully absorb their benefits. As well as therapeutic herbs, rasayana includes foods such as milk, ghee, and honey.

"Not for yourself, not for gain, but solely for the good of humanity should you treat your patients."

CHARAKA

Ayurveda's six criteria
of therapeutic properties encompass the effects a substance has on you from first taste to digestion and absorption.

HOME REMEDIES

FOR COMMON AILMENTS

*"The greater part of the treatment
of an Ayurvedic practitioner
is by medicinal herbs."*

SWAMI SIVANANDA

TREATING COMMON AILMENTS BY DOSHA

In Ayurveda, the dosha imbalances causing a disease are treated as well as the disease itself. For this reason it is important to consider dominant or elavated dosha(s) when choosing remedies.

Ailments as imbalances

Herbs and spices are essential to support the body's functions according to Ayurveda, and so Ayurvedic home remedies use high dosages of these ingredients to correct imbalances in the body.

Elevation of any of the three doshas can cause any disease, but many diseases are commonly caused by the elevation of one or more specific dosha(s) (see right). How a disease presents itself is dependent on the constitution of the individual. By examining the symptoms of a disease in a specific person, an experienced Ayurvedic practitioner can determine which dosha(s) and qualities are involved, and prescribe a suitable remedy for that person.

Many common ailments cause similar problems in people of all constitutions; in these cases, there are general remedies that can be used. For example, the term "common cold" already points to the quality "cold", therefore any remedy that is heating will help.

Choosing the right remedy

In the remedy lists that follow, some remedies are listed as "for all doshas" if they are suitable for everyone. The other remedies will be listed as only for one or two doshas, this means they are only meant for those whose constitution is mainly made up of those doshas (eg. if it says for pitta and kapha only, it should not be taken by someone with dominant or elevated vata). If the home remedies in this chapter do not help you, we advise that you seek professional medical advice.

VATA

If vata is dominant in your constitution, or you have elevated vata, be careful to avoid anything that increases dryness, lightness, movement and cold, and is pungent, bitter, and astringent as this will elevate vata further.

AILMENTS

Vata is most commonly involved in bone and joint problems, common cold, heart disease, diseases of the colon, urinary and genital tract, and any type of trauma.

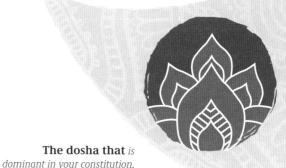

The dosha that is
dominant in your constitution,
or that is imbalanced in your body,
will affect the symptoms you have
and remedies you should use.

KAPHA

If kapha is dominant in your constitution, or you have elevated kapha, be careful to avoid anything that is sweet, salty, and sour, and increases heaviness, cold, oiliness, moisture, and stickiness, as this will elevate kapha further.

AILMENTS

Kapha is most commonly involved in diseases of the respiratory tract and stomach, common cold, diabetes, slow metabolism and any condition where there is heaviness, increased mucous, blockage, swelling, and excess tissue.

THE HEALING
POWER OF PLANTS

Ayurveda holds medicinal plants in high regard because they contain the cosmic energy of the sun (the greatest-known source of healing power in Ayurvedic philosophy) and store the healing potency of moonlight. Medicinal plants convert valuable inorganic earth salts, chemicals, and minerals into organic matter, making them more readily accessible to human physiology. They are made up of the five elements (earth, water, fire, air, and ether) and affect every cell of the body.

IMPORTANT NOTE

Seeking professional medical advice will aid the diagnosis of ailments and the prescription of remedies and dosages.

When using the remedies in this book, follow the preparation and dosage instructions carefully.

If any remedy appears to make the ailment worse, or fails to improve an ailment after 3 days, stop using it and seek professional medical advice.

If you are pregnant or treating a child, always seek professional medical advice before using any remedy.

Reduce dosages by ½ when treating a child.

PITTA

If pitta is dominant in your constitution, or you have elevated pitta, be careful to avoid anything that increases heat, lightness, oiliness, and is pungent, sour, and stimulating, as this will elevate pitta further. Use long pepper instead of ginger or black pepper.

AILMENTS

Pitta is most commonly involved in diseases of the skin, blood, eyes, liver, stomach, and small intestine, and any condition with increased acidity.

HOW TO PREPARE
HOME REMEDIES

Many of the remedies described in this book are simple to use. Instructions on how to prepare and administer more complex or less familiar remedies are given here.

MEASUREMENTS

Throughout the chapter, small quantities are given in teaspoons for ease.

- **¼ tsp** 1g (1/28oz)
- **½ tsp** 2g (1/14oz)
- **Level tsp** 3g (3/28oz)
- **Heaped tsp** 5g (1/6oz)

DECOCTIONS

This is an extract made by boiling herbs or spices in water. Plant chemicals diffuse into the water and become concentrated as the liquid boils. Decoctions can be consumed, applied locally, or used for a bath.

1 **Mix 60g (2oz) ground herb** or spice with 1 litre (1¾ pints) water. If you are using whole or solid parts, double the quantity of the herb.

2 **Boil until only** 250ml (9fl oz) liquid remains, then strain the liquid and discard the solid parts of the herb or spice.

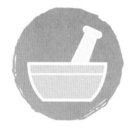

PASTES

This smooth mixture is made by combining ground spices or ground dried herbs with a liquid such as water or oil. A paste should be applied locally, and left in place for 20–30 minutes before being washed off.

1 **Mix 1 part ground** spices or ground dried herbs with ¼ part water or ½ part oil.

2 **You can keep the paste** in a jar for 24 hours. Pastes are most effective when used immediately.

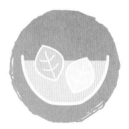

COLD EXTRACTS

A cold extract is the filtered water of a herb or spice soaked in water overnight. It can be consumed or applied locally.

1 **Use 1 part ground herb** or spice with 8 parts water. (If you are using whole or solid parts, double the quantity of the herb).

2 **Steep in cold water** overnight or for at least 8 hours, then strain the liquid and discard the herb.

"Ayurveda is a perfect science of life and consists of a body of most remarkable knowledge on medicinal herbs and therapeutic roots."

SWAMI SIVANANDA

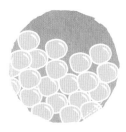

PILLS & LOZENGES

These are small, solid balls made from ground herbs or spices and a sticky substance. Pills should be swallowed, and lozenges sucked or chewed.

1 **Combine 1 part ground herbs** or spices to ¼ part honey, ghee, or oil.

2 **Roll on a dry clean surface** until you have a solid pill or lozenge.

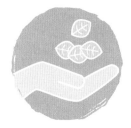

POULTICES

Made from herbs, poultices are applied locally to the skin and held in place with a bandage for 1 hour or more. Either use fresh, whole leaves, or make the leaves into a paste (see below). If using whole leaves, skip straight to step 2.

1 **Crush fresh leaves** and/or solid parts of a plant to a pulp in a mortar. Add a small amount of water to bind the leaves into a paste if necessary. If using dried leaves, boil them in water for 5 minutes to unlock the active ingredients. Then drain the boiling water and crush the leaves into a paste.

2 **Apply a thick** layer of poultice (paste or whole leaves) locally. Then cover with gauze and secure with a bandage.

3 **Leave the poultice** in place for 1–2 hours, or overnight if possible. Then remove the coverings and wash the affected area.

AYURVEDIC INGREDIENTS

According to the ancient scripture by Charaka, Ayurvedic principles can be applied to any plant with known therapeutic properties, but plants grown locally are most effective.

Remedies in this chapter use some plants from the ancient Indian scriptures. Most can now be found throughout the world in good supermarkets, Indian food shops, health-food shops, or online.

- **Tulsi** – this plant is also known as holy basil. The leaves can be used to make a tea, or the juice from them extracted.
- **Long pepper (pippali)** – rare in European cuisine, it is widely available from Indian food shops.
- **Psyllium husk** – this powder is made from the outer coating of seeds from the psyllium plant.

REMEDIES FOR
COMMON AILMENTS

This section includes a variety of common acute and chronic ailments. The remedies given relieve specific symptoms and are not intended as a substitute for professional treatment of chronic disease. It is best to use one remedy at a time for a specific condition.

Anaemia

These remedies should be used alongside professional treatment.

FOR ALL DOSHAS

- Boil 100g (3½oz) rice with 2 tsp fenugreek seeds, ¼ tsp salt, and 1 tbsp ghee. Eat once or twice a day, ideally for breakfast and lunch. Omit the salt if you have high blood pressure.
- Take ½ tsp turmeric with 1 tbsp cane sugar and 1 tsp ghee three times a day.

Anxiety

Anxiety at times of stress is normal, and can be alleviated with these remedies. Sustained anxiety requires professional treatment.

FOR VATA & PITTA ONLY

- Boil 200ml (7fl oz) milk with 1 tsp cane sugar, 1 tsp fennel seeds, and 2 threads saffron. Drink the mixture warm, taking 100ml (3½fl oz) twice daily.

FOR KAPHA ONLY

- The best anxiety remedy for dominant or elevated kapha is physical exercise.

Bad breath

Mostly caused by poor oral hygiene, persistent bad breath may require professional medical advice.

FOR ALL DOSHAS

- Chew 2 cloves up to three times a day.

- Boil 1 cup (240ml/8fl oz) water with 1 tsp ground cardamom and 1 tsp ground cinnamon and drink three times a day.

Cholesterol, high

These remedies aim to help lower cholesterol. Seek professional medical advice before using them.

FOR ALL DOSHAS

- Take ½ tsp fenugreek seeds daily.

FOR VATA & KAPHA ONLY

- Use chilli generously in your meals.

Diabetes

These remedies aim to help lower blood sugar. Seek professional medical advice before using them. If you have poorly controlled diabetes, avoid honey.

FOR ALL DOSHAS

- Drink 1 tsp lemon juice with ½ tsp honey three times a day.
- Make a decoction of 1 tbsp ground turmeric, 3 bay leaves, and 1 tbsp fenugreek seeds and drink ½ cup (120ml/4fl oz) before each meal; or take these herbs in the same proportions with honey before each meal.

DIET

- Eat spinach, lettuce, cabbage, tomatoes, coconut, leafy vegetables, and sour fruit.
- Avoid eating rice, sugar, sweet fruits, all starchy foods.

YOGA

- Practise deep breathing, sun salutation, shoulderstand, and forward bend.

Earache

Earaches often heal in a few days without treatment. These remedies help alleviate pain and speed recovery.

FOR ALL DOSHAS

- Press the juice from fresh ginger and apply a drop to the ear as needed.
- Apply a drop of tulsi oil, marjoram oil, or dill oil to the edge of the ear canal as needed.

Fatigue

Sustained tiredness can be caused by lack of sleep, stress, or a medical condition. These remedies aim to help you feel more energized. If fatigue persists, seek professional medical attention.

FOR ALL DOSHAS

- Peel coriander seeds by rolling them in kitchen paper, and use the peeled seeds to make a tea. Drink 1 cup (240ml/8fl oz) as needed.

FOR VATA & PITTA ONLY

- Boil 100ml (3½fl oz) milk with 1 tsp almond butter, 1 tsp cane sugar, and a pinch saffron and ground ginger. Drink one or two times a day. This is helpful if you have had weight loss.

Fever

If a fever (constant or remittent) lasts for more than 3 days, seek medical advice, or ealier if the fever worsens or is joined by other symptoms (such as vomiting). Seek medical advice for fever in children.

FOR ALL DOSHAS

- Eat or chew 3 black peppercorns, 5–10 basil leaves, and 5 neem leaves (ideally fresh) up to three times a day.
- Boil 3–4 cloves in 1 litre (1¾ pints) water for 30 minutes and drink in small sips throughout the day.

Headache

These remedies aim to alleviate pain from minor headaches. If headaches return regularly, seek professional medical advice.

FOR ALL DOSHAS

- Drink 1 cup (240ml/8fl oz) hot water with 2 tbsp lemon juice in the morning and before going to bed.
- Drink lime juice sweetened with cane sugar and ¼ tsp ground cardamom and a pinch black pepper three times a day.
- Apply camphor oil to the head as needed.

FOR VATA & KAPHA ONLY

- Apply 1 tbsp grated ginger mixed with 1 tsp honey to the tender area as needed.
- Apply a paste of ground black cardamom or a black pepper poultice to the forehead as needed.

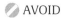

AVOID

- Drinking black tea and coffee
- Working too hard or late at night
- Straining the eyes
- Stress.

Heat & hot flushes

Those with dominant or elevated pitta can feel overheated, and should take care to keep cool (physically and emotionally), especially in summer. These remedies are also helpful for hot flushes during menopause.

FOR ALL DOSHAS

- Make a decoction of 2 tsp fried ground fenugreek seeds and drink 1 cup (240ml/8fl oz) up to three times a day. For vata and pitta, add 1 tsp ghee.
- Massage the body with dried ground fennel seeds.

FOR VATA ONLY

- Take 1–2 tsp pure ghee a day.

FOR PITTA ONLY

- Take 3–4 tsp pure ghee a day.

Heat in the head

This is a feeling of heat that only affects the head.

FOR ALL DOSHAS

- Rub castor oil onto the soles of the feet at night.

Insomnia

Use these remedies to help you get to sleep and stay asleep at night.

FOR VATA & PITTA ONLY

- Boil 100ml (3½fl oz) milk with ½ tsp nutmeg, ½ tsp almond milk, and ½ tsp cane sugar. Drink 30 minutes before going to bed.

FOR KAPHA ONLY

- The best insomnia remedy for kapha consitution or elevated kapha is physical exercise.

Migraine

Migraines are headaches with throbbing on one side of the head. They can cause nausea, vomitting, and sensitivity to light and sound.

FOR ALL DOSHAS

- Mix 2 threads saffron with 1 tsp ghee, and apply into the nostrils up to three times a day.

FOR VATA & KAPHA ONLY

- Apply a heated mixture of 2 tbsp sesame oil with 1 tsp cardamom and ½ tsp ground cinnamon to the forehead.

Nosebleed

Seek immediate professional medical treatment for nosebleeds caused by a head injury, with excessive bleeding, or those lasting more than 20 minutes.

FOR ALL DOSHAS

- Carefully apply juice of fresh coriander leaves to the nostrils with your little finger.
- Make a paste of ground basil seeds and carefully apply into the nostrils with your little finger.

Urinary tract infection

See a doctor if your symptoms don't improve in a few days.

FOR ALL DOSHAS

- Drink 4 tsp of a decoction of tulsi seeds twice a day.
- Take ¼–½ tsp ground green cardamom in 1 tsp ghee up to three times a day.
- Drink 1 cup (240ml/8fl oz) cold extract or decoction of equal parts fennel and coriander seeds, or eat 1 tsp fresh coriander up to three times a day.

Weight loss

Weight loss can be caused by a variety of problems. Seek professional medical advice for serious weight loss (more than 5% body weight) if you have not had a recent period of stress and/or an eating disorder.

FOR ALL DOSHAS

- Mix 2 tsp tulsi leaf juice with 1 tsp honey and take three times a day for at least a month.

REMEDIES FOR **RESPIRATORY TRACT AILMENTS**

These remedies will help to alleviate symptoms of ailments affecting the respiratory tract. For acute conditions that involve phelgm and mucous, follow the kapha diet by avoiding kapha-elevating foods (for more information, see pp.80–83).

Asthma

This condition can be caused by any dosha, but kapha is most commonly involved. These remedies add relief to conventional treatment.

FOR ALL DOSHAS

- Make pills (see p.203) using 2 tsp ground cloves and 1 tsp honey. Take 2 pills three times a day.
- Mix 1 tsp tulsi leaf juice with ½ tsp ground black pepper and drink 2 tsp three times a day.
- Take 1 cup (240ml/8fl oz) orange or lemon juice with 1 tsp honey.

Bronchitis

Seek professional medical advice if your cough lasts longer than 3 weeks, you have a fever for more than 3 days, you have chest pains or difficulty breathing, or you have repeated bouts of bronchitis.

FOR ALL DOSHAS

- Chew on mint leaves.
- Apply a poultice made with mustard seeds to the chest. For vata and kapha, leave it on as long as needed. Those with dominant or elavated pitta should wash off after 10 minutes.

🖐 **DIET**

- Follow a kapha diet (see pp.80–83).

Common cold

Rest, sleep, and hydration are best. These remedies will help support the healing process and alleviate symptoms. Only treat children after seeking medical advice and under medical supervision.

FOR ALL DOSHAS

- In the early stages, drink tulsi tea or ground ginger and coriander tea as needed.
- Eat 2–3 dates, and drink 1 tsp lemon juice in warm water twice a day.

FOR VATA & KAPHA ONLY

- Steep 1 tsp ground black cardamom in 1 cup (240ml/8fl oz) hot water and drink it up to three times a day.

FOR PITTA ONLY

- Steep 1 tsp ground green cardamom in 1 cup (240ml/8fl oz) hot water and drink it up to three times a day.

🖐 **DIET**

- Follow a kapha diet (see pp.80–83).

✋ **AVOID**

- Exposure to wind and cold, particularly of the head.

🧍 **CHILDREN**

- Drink tulsi tea up to three times a day.

Cough

Rest and hydration are best. These remedies aim to support the healing process and alleviate symptoms. If your cough lasts longer than 3 weeks, seek professional medical advice; children should be assessed after 1 week. Only treat children after seeking medical advice and under medical supervision.

Productive cough

These remedies aim to alleviate coughs that produce mucous or phlegm.

FOR ALL DOSHAS

- Take 1 tsp honey three times a day, with 1 tsp lemon juice or tulsi leaf juice. Honey is drying and should only be taken as long as the cough is productive. If required, 1 tsp licorice, salt, or sugar counteracts its dryness.
- Make a decoction of long pepper and cinnamon. For vata or pitta, add ½ tsp cane sugar. Drink 30ml (2 tbsp) two to three times a day.
- Make a lozenge (see p.203) out of 1 tsp honey with 2 tsp ground cloves, or 1 tsp ground ginger and 1 tsp ground green cardamom. Take as needed.

FOR VATA & KAPHA ONLY

- Take 1 tsp honey with 1 tsp black pepper three times a day.

FOR PITTA ONLY

- Take 1 tsp honey with ½ tsp long pepper three times a day.

Non-productive cough

These remedies aim to alleviate dry coughs.

FOR ALL DOSHAS

- Mix 1 tbsp fresh ginger juice with 1 tsp raw cane sugar and drink. Perform a steam inhalation afterwards (lean over a bowel of hot water and cover the head with a towel for 20–30 minutes).
- Mix 1 tsp ground fennel seeds, ½ tsp licorice, and ½ tsp rock candy. Add 1 tsp of the mixture to 1 tsp honey and take three times a day.

FOR VATA

- Dissolve 1 flake rock salt in your mouth as many times a day as you feel comfortable. Do not use if you have high blood pressure.

CHILDREN

- Heat 4–8 threads of saffron in 1 cup (240ml/8fl oz) of milk, and divide into three to four portions. Use in single portions throughout the day.

Mouth ulcers

Ulcers can be uncomfortable, but generally clear up themselves with time. These remedies aim to soothe them and speed up recovery. Try one of these remedies at a time.

FOR ALL DOSHAS

- Apply a honey or almond paste up to three times a day.
- Gargle fresh coriander leaf juice up to three times a day.
- Gargle fresh mint juice up to three times a day.

Respiratory tract infections

These remedies give relief to respiratory tract infections

ranging from the common cold to bronchitis.

FOR ALL DOSHAS

- Boil 2 tbsp garden cress seeds with 1 tsp long pepper and 1 tsp tulsi, and mix with 1 tsp cane sugar. Filter and drink 120ml (4fl oz) up to three times a day.

FOR VATA & PITTA ONLY

- Take ⅛ tsp black pepper with ½ tsp sugar, or, for pitta, with ½ tsp ghee.

FOR KAPHA ONLY

- Take ⅛ tsp black pepper with 1 tsp honey.

DIET

- Follow a kapha diet (see pp.80–83).

Runny nose

A runny nose is often associated with a cold. These remedies aim to alleviate symptoms. Seek professional advice if a runny nose persists to the extent that it is affecting your quality of life.

FOR ALL DOSHAS

- Crush 1 tsp caraway seeds in a mortar, put in a cloth and inhale the essential oils as needed.
- Heat ½ tsp ground turmeric in 1 cup (240ml/8fl oz) milk and drink twice a day.

Sinus headache

This is felt as a dull, throbbing pain in the upper face. It is often caused by a cold. If you have particularly a bad headache, or one that lasts a day or more, seek professional medical advice.

FOR ALL DOSHAS

- Inhale a pinch dry ground ginger or eucalyptus or cinnamon oil in each nostril.

FOR VATA & KAPHA ONLY

- Apply a paste of ground ginger or a mixture of equal parts cinnamon,

black pepper, and warm water to the forehead and temples.

DIET

- Follow a kapha diet (see pp.80–83).

Sore throat

Symptoms usually subside in less than a week. These remedies aim to help soothe pain and speed recovery. Seek professional medical attention if a sore throat lasts for longer than a week, or if you also have a very high temperature.

FOR ALL DOSHAS

- Gargle hot water mixed with either ½ tsp rock salt or 1 tbsp lemon juice.

FOR VATA & KAPHA ONLY

- Gargle tea made from ½ tsp chilli.

Sore throat with hoarseness

FOR ALL DOSHAS

- Make a lozenge (see p.203) using 1 tsp honey and 2 tsp long pepper, and take as needed.
- Drink ¼ tsp turmeric in 1 cup (240ml/8fl oz) hot milk with ½–1 tsp cane sugar.

Voice loss

This usually heals within a couple of weeks, and these remedies will speed the process. Seek professional medical advice if it persists for more than 2 weeks, if you find it too painful to swallow food, or you get repeated bouts.

FOR ALL DOSHAS

- To protect your vocal cords from strain, make a lozenge (see p.203) of ¼ tsp ground ginger mixed with honey.
- If your voice or throat is hoarse, use cane sugar and water instead of honey. Gargle the mixture with 1 tbsp sesame oil.

REMEDIES FOR **DIGESTIVE TRACT AILMENTS**

There is no physical health without a healthy digestive tract – this is seen in the importance of agni (digestive fire) and digestion in the creation of dhatus (tissues) and ojas (immunity) in the body (see pp.26–27). These remedies bring quick relief to many minor ailments.

Appetite loss

These remedies are intended for those who have a loss of appetite when food is still required, such as in times of stress. Loss of appetite due to disease is a serious problem, and should be treated only under the supervision of a medical professional.

FOR ALL DOSHAS

- Have a pinch rock salt with 1 tbsp lemon juice or ½ cup (120ml/4fl oz) buttermilk up to three times a day. (Omit salt if you have high blood pressure.)
- Drink 1 tbsp lemon or ginger juice with ½ tsp honey up to three times a day.
- Take ½ tsp black pepper with raw cane sugar up to three times a day. Drink a glass of warm water after taking the pepper.

Colitis or irritable colon

This remedy can be used in addition to professional medical treatment and dietary advice.

FOR ALL DOSHAS

- Mix equal parts sesame oil, ghee, turmeric, and honey and take 2 tsp three times a day.

Constipation

This should be corrected as soon as possible. Alongside a proper diet, these remedies will help.

FOR ALL DOSHAS

- Drink a glass of hot water early in the morning; for vata and kapha, add a pinch rock salt. (Omit salt if you have high blood pressure.)
- Soak 1 part psyllium husk in 6 parts water and drink ½ cup (120ml/ 4fl oz) three to four times a day.
- To support peristalsis, soak dill seeds in water overnight and take 1 tsp seeds before every meal.

FOR VATA & PITTA ONLY

- Drink 1 cup (240ml/8fl oz) aloe vera juice in the morning and evening.
- Before going to bed, drink 1 cup (240ml/8fl oz) lukewarm water or warmed milk mixed with 3 tsp melted ghee.

🍽 **DIET**

- Increase the amount of vegetables that you eat.
- Figs, plums, raisins, prunes, dates, grapes, leafy vegetables, licorice, linseed, and molasses are all beneficial.
- Drink buttermilk.

🧘 **YOGA**

- Practise deep breathing, sun salutation, shoulderstand, forward bend, and cobra.

Diarrhoea

These remedies support medical treatment and help maintain good agni (digestive fire). Seek professional medical advice if you have no appetite and experience weight loss, if your stool is dark and smelly (this may indicate bleeding), or the diarrhoea doesn't go away within 3 days. Always seek professional medical advice before treating a baby or child, and only use these remedies under professional medical supervision.

FOR ALL DOSHAS

- Take ½ tsp ground ginger with ½ tsp caraway seeds and 1 tsp jaggery twice a day; or take 1 tsp cane sugar in 1 tbsp lemon juice twice a day.
- Take ½ tsp ground coriander, ¼ tsp ground cumin, a pinch ginger and a pinch salt in 1 cup (240ml/8fl oz) warm water throughout the day.
- To support stool formation, soak 1 tsp psyllium husk in 1 cup (240ml/8fl oz) water and drink three times a day.

🍽 **DIET**

- Eat walnuts, poppy seeds, soaked fenugreek seeds.
- Drink buttermilk and pomegranate juice.

👶 **CHILDREN**

- Give the affected child a pinch nutmeg and ¼ tsp ground ginger in some ghee.

Flatulence & bloating

This is most often a sign that vata is elevated, so these remedies are intended to help pacify vata.

FOR VATA & KAPHA ONLY

- Take ½ tsp ground ajwain, ½ tsp ground ginger, and a pinch black salt in 1 cup (240ml/8fl oz) warm water before every meal. (Omit salt if you have high blood pressure.)

DIET

- Long pepper, lemon, coriander, fresh or ground ginger, mint, black pepper, fenugreek seeds, fennel, nutmeg, tulsi, turmeric, ajwain seeds, aniseed, caraway seeds, cardamom, chamomile, cinnamon, cloves, cumin, bay leaves, and dill seeds are all beneficial.

BABIES

- Apply warm dill seed oil or castor oil around the navel.

Gastritis

These remedies can help reduce stomach acidity and increase agni (digestive fire). Seek professional medical advice if symptoms last more than 3 days, or if the pain is worsening.

FOR ALL DOSHAS

- Make a pill (see p.203) from ¼ tsp ground ginger, 1 tsp ghee and 1 tsp jaggery, and take it 15–30 minutes before every meal.

FOR VATA & KAPHA ONLY

- Eat 1 tsp ajwain immediately after meals.

FOR PITTA ONLY

- Eat 1 tsp turmeric after every meal.

DIET

- Eat carrots, coconut, soaked fenugreek seeds, leafy vegetables, and mung dhal.
- Drink lemon juice in warm water.

- Avoid eating sour fruit, pungent spices, and yogurt.

Gastritis with stomach pain

Sometimes gastritis occurs with stomach cramps. In such cases, use these remedies to alleviate pain.

FOR ALL DOSHAS

- Drink a decoction of ground cloves. Clove reduces inflammation and acts as a local anaesthetic.

Heartburn or acid reflux

Try using the following remedies when you have an empty stomach and after meals. Seek professional medical advice if you experience persistent heartburn over 3 weeks.

FOR ALL DOSHAS

- Drink 1 cup (240ml/8fl oz) pomegranate juice mixed with 1 tsp honey up to three times a day.
- Take 1 tsp ground cumin with honey in equal parts up to three times a day.

Indigestion & weak agni (digestive fire)

Try these remedies on a daily basis to increase your wellbeing. See also diet for agni on pp.84–85. Seek professional medical advice if you get indigestion regularly or if the pain is worsening.

FOR ALL DOSHAS

- Drink 1 tbsp lemon and 1 tsp ginger juice in 1 cup (240ml/8fl oz) warm water with 1 tsp honey every morning.
- Eat a bit of ginger-raisin chutney (see p.110) immediately before every meal.

FOR VATA & PITTA ONLY

- Chew ¼ tsp coriander seeds.

FOR VATA & KAPHA ONLY

- Eat ½ tsp fresh ginger with a pinch

---

salt immediately before each meal. (Omit salt if you have high blood pressure.)
- After heavy meals, drink a black pepper decoction.

FOR PITTA ONLY

- After a heavy meal, drink a long pepper decoction, or take 1 tsp ground cumin boiled in 1 cup (240ml/8fl oz) buttermilk with a small amount of vegetable oil and a pinch rock salt.

FOR PITTA & KAPHA ONLY

- Eat a bit of ground long pepper with honey immediately before every meal.

DIET

- Use plenty of spices when cooking meals. For vata and kapha, black cardamom is especially beneficial. For pitta, bitter herbs, such as turmeric, are beneficial.

YOGA

- Practise asanas and 3 minutes of deep breathing each day.

Nausea

Severe nausea and vomiting require immediate professional medical attention. These remedies can be used in cases of mild nausea.

FOR ALL DOSHAS

- Eat ½ tsp fresh ginger mixed with 1 tbsp lemon juice and a pinch rock salt as needed, but no more than once every 10 minutes. (Omit salt if you have high blood pressure.)
- Drink a strong tea or decoction of caraway seeds, coriander seeds (can also be chewed), fennel, or mint as needed.

REMEDIES FOR AILMENTS OF THE
EYES, HAIR, SKIN, AND TEETH

This section includes ailments that affect the eyes, hair, skin, and teeth. Most remedies here are intended to alleviate the symptoms of the listed ailments. Some, such as many for the eyes and teeth, are general practices to improve general health and function.

Eyes

The eyes have a strong connection to the dosha pitta. The following remedies can be used to help improve vision.

FOR ALL DOSHAS

- Soak 2 threads saffron in 30ml (1fl oz) rosewater overnight and use the solution as eye drops.
- Drink 2–4 tsp fresh fennel juice daily.

FOR VATA & PITTA ONLY

- Take 1 tsp ghee mixed with ¼ tsp chickpea flour and ¼ tsp cane sugar.

Conjunctivitis

Take these remedies alongside conventional medical treatments. Seek professional medical advice if symptoms persist for more than 2 days.

FOR ALL DOSHAS

- Boil 1 part ground turmeric with 10 parts water, let it cool, then soak a cotton ball in it and apply to the eye.
- Steep 1 tsp ground cumin in 1 cup (240ml/8fl oz) hot water. Apply the solution to the eye in an eye bath cup.
- Apply a decoction of coriander or juice of fresh coriander to the eyes using a cotton ball.
- Apply a drop of honey to the eyes two to three times a day using a cotton ball.

Hair loss

Temporary hair loss can be caused by stress, illness, or treatment. These remedies aim to help alleviate hair loss. Seek professional medical advice if you have sudden hair loss, are losing hair in clumps, or your head itches or burns.

FOR ALL DOSHAS

- Make a paste from fenugreek leaves and apply to the scalp.
- Make a paste from roasted, ground fenugreek seeds and apply to the scalp. Wash off after 30–60 minutes.

Skin

Skin, blood, and pitta have a close connection. Anything that is bitter and cooling is often helpful, as these pacify pitta. Fenugreek, ground turmeric, and neem can be taken orally or applied locally to help alleviate skin problems.

Abscess

These remedies are intended to ripen an abscess or pimple and should be used on the advice of a medical professional.

FOR ALL DOSHAS

- Apply a poultice made from black pepper to the affected area.

- Apply a paste of dill leaves to the affected area, or slowly heat 5–10 dill leaves in 1 cup (240ml/8fl oz) sesame oil and apply.

Acne

These remedies aim to alleviate minor acne. Seek professional medical advice if you think you have severe acne.

FOR ALL DOSHAS

- Apply 1 tsp ground turmeric mixed with ¼ tsp lemon juice or ½ tsp honey to the affected area.
- Make a cumin paste and then apply as a face mask.
- Apply a paste of crushed caraway seeds with water or sesame oil.
- Apply a paste of nutmeg, ground turmeric, and black pepper.

Complexion

These remedies are intended to improve complexion and rejuvenate your skin.

FOR ALL DOSHAS

- Make a paste from soaked fenugreek seeds and use it as a face mask.
- Apply milk mixed with a pinch nutmeg to the skin up to three times a day.
- To clear skin, add some saffron to skin lotion or apply a poultice made from saffron.

Dry, cracked skin

These remedies aim to alleviate dry skin. If problems persist, seek professional medical advice.

FOR ALL DOSHAS

- Apply ½ tsp ground turmeric in 1 tsp ghee or castor oil.

Hives

Rashes usually subside in 1–2 days. Seek professional medical advice if a rash persists for more than 3 days.

FOR ALL DOSHAS

- Take 1 tsp ajwain seeds mixed with 1 tsp cane sugar after two of your daily meals.
- Boil 1 tsp mint and 2 tsp cane sugar in water, and drink 1 cup (240ml/8fl oz) up to three times a day.

Insect bites & stings

Usually bites and stings take only a few hours or days to heal. Seek professional medical advice if a sting covers 5cm (2in) or more, if it becomes infected, or if it doesn't improve after 3 days.

FOR ALL DOSHAS

- Use tulsi oil, eucalyptus oil, and neem oil as mosquito repellents.
- Rub bites with tulsi leaves.
- Mix 1 tsp ground cumin with 1 tsp ghee and apply the mixture to the bite. This reduces pain, swelling, and counteracts the toxin.
- For wasp or bee stings, apply a poultice of crushed bay leaves.

Itching

Itchy skin can be caused by any of the doshas, most frequently kapha, then vata, and, least often, pitta.

VATA & KAPHA

- Apply mustard oil or a poultice made from mustard seeds.

Skin irritation or rashes

Rashes usually subside in 1–2 days. Seek professional medical advice if a rash persists for more than 3 days, or if it is accompanied by fever.

FOR ALL DOSHAS

- Apply aloe vera gel with ground turmeric or a paste made from ground turmeric to the rash; remove after it dries. Do this three to four times a day. (It is best to use aloe vera gel with no added citric acid, as the acid counteracts the cooling quality of the aloe.)
- Apply a wet poultice made with ajwain paste to the affected area.
- Apply a paste made of fresh garden cress leaf to the affected area.
- Apply a paste of ground cumin or add 2 tbsp cumin to your bath water.
- Apply a paste made from ground green cardamom seeds.

FOR VATA & KAPHA ONLY

- Apply a warm paste of ground black cardamom and water, do not apply to the face.

Teeth

Oral hygiene is seen as an integral part of daily hygiene in Ayurveda. Use the following remedies to keep your teeth healthy.

FOR ALL DOSHAS

- Chew neem leaves daily (neem is an antiseptic).
- Eat a bit of sour food at the end of every meal (the acid helps to keep your teeth clean).
- Rinse your mouth with salt water every morning.
- Rinse your mouth with water after eating sweets or sugary foods.
- Clean your teeth with neem sticks.
- Practise oil pulling (see p.34).

FOR VATA & KAPHA ONLY

- Massage your gums daily with mustard oil mixed with salt.

Toothache

These remedies are mainly antiseptics and will relieve pain caused by tootache. Seek professional medical treatment if toothache lasts more than 2 days.

FOR ALL DOSHAS

- Chew 2 cloves up to three times a day.
- Apply clove oil on a cotton swab to the affected area. (Warning! Do not apply for too long, as it can cause ulcers.)
- Brush teeth with ground black pepper or Trikatu (a mixture of equal parts ground ginger, black pepper, and long pepper). Alternatively, make a decoction of Trikatu and gargle it.

FOR VATA & KAPHA ONLY

- Gargle mustard oil with a pinch salt.
- Gargle a decoction of black cardamom.

REMEDIES FOR **TRAUMA AND MUSCULOSKELETAL AILMENTS**

Vata is aggravated by trauma, and pain is a vata function; kapha is most often involved in swelling; pitta causes redness and heat. Many of these conditions require immediate professional medical attention. If you are unsure, always seek professional medical advice.

Body pain (general)

If pain is severe, or persists for more than 3 days, seek immediate professional medical advice.

FOR ALL DOSHAS

- For external pain, apply marjoram oil or ghee, nutmeg paste, or water with a warm paste made from crushed mustard seeds up to three times a day.
- Massage the affected area with a mixture of equal parts camphor oil and mustard oil, or ground fenugreek with equal parts mustard oil and cinnamon oil up to three times a day.

FOR VATA AND KAPHA

- For internal pain, take ⅓ tsp black cardamom, ⅓ tsp ground turmeric and ⅓ tsp black pepper in 1 tsp ghee up to three times a day.

FOR PITTA AND KAPHA

- For internal pain, take ⅓ tsp green cardamom, ⅓ tsp turmeric, and ⅓ tsp black pepper in honey up to three times a day.

Bone fractures & osteoporosis

Always seek professional medical advice for these conditions. In both cases, there is loss of the bone dhatu (tissue). The ginger ensures that agni (digestive fire) is strong enough to produce new, healthy dhatu.

FOR ALL DOSHAS

- Drink 1 cup (240ml/8fl oz) warm milk with 1 tsp licorice and 1 tsp ginger twice a day.

Burns (minor)

These remedies are intended only for minor burns, and should only be used after the affected area has been held under cold, running water for 10 minutes. For more serious burns seek immediate professional medical advice. Honey is drying and cooling, while ghee and fenugreek leaves are cooling. This makes them effective at alleviating pain and helping a burn to heal.

FOR ALL DOSHAS

- Apply honey to the burn as needed.
- Apply a paste of fenugreek leaves to the burn as needed.
- Apply ghee to the burn as needed.

Lumbago & sciatica

These remedies aim to ease lower-back and leg pain. Seek professional medical advice if symptoms don't improve after 3 weeks, if pain worsens, or if it stops you fulfilling daily tasks and responsibilities.

FOR ALL DOSHAS

- Apply a poultice made from chilli powder as needed.

- Apply 1 tsp ground cinnamon and 1 tsp ground ginger heated in 1 cup (240ml/8fl oz) sesame oil as needed.

Numbness in the extremities

These remedies are intended to be used alongside professional medical treatment.

FOR ALL DOSHAS

- Apply fresh mint paste or mint oil.

FOR VATA & KAPHA ONLY

- Apply mustard oil mixed with ground chilli up to twice a day – make sure to wash off properly afterwards.

Osteoarthritis

These remedies are intended to alleviate pain and swelling. Always seek professional medical advice and use these remedies under professional medical supervision.

FOR ALL DOSHAS

- Mix 2 tsp garden cress seeds with 1 tsp lemon juice, crush in a mortar and apply the paste.
- Mix 2 tsp garden cress with 1 tsp lemon juice and apply the mixture to the affected joint.
- Massage the affected part of the body with castor oil.

Rheumatism & rheumatoid arthritis

These remedies are intended to alleviate pain. Both conditions indicate the prescence of ama (toxins), so be sure to also do practices that digest ama and strengthen agni (see pp.56–57).

FOR ALL DOSHAS

- Take 1 tsp ground ginger in 1 cup (240ml/8fl oz) yogurt or milk curd up to three times a day.
- Boil 1 tsp ground garden cress seeds in 100ml (3½fl oz) milk and take three times a day.
- Boil and crush dill seeds in a mortar, then use them to make a paste. Apply the paste to the affected area.
- Apply a warm paste of soaked marjoram, or take a bath containing a marjoram decoction.
- Take ½ tsp ground ginger with 1 tsp honey or ½ tsp castor oil three times a day after meals.
- Massage the affected area with equal parts castor oil and clove oil.

FOR VATA AND PITTA

- Take ½ tsp ground ginger with 1 tsp ghee three times a day after meals.

FOR VATA AND KAPHA

- Take ¼–½ tsp ground chilli with honey up to three times a day.
- Massage the affected area with castor oil mixed with chilli as needed.

Sprains

Swelling is often a sign of kapha, which can be alleviated by heat and dryness. Any trauma aggravates vata, which can be alleviated by heat and stability. Seek professional medical advice if you are unable to move the joint, if the limb gives way when you try to use it, or if pain is particularly intense.

FOR ALL DOSHAS

- Apply a cold water pack until the

swelling goes down. For painful sprains, apply a hot water pack.
- Massage the affected area with bay leaf oil or castor oil.

Swelling & pain in the joints & limbs

Pain indicates the involvement of vata, while swelling indicates kapha. Anything that strengthens agni will be helpful (see pp.56–57). If symptoms don't improve after 3 days, seek professional medical advice.

FOR ALL DOSHAS

- Take 1 tsp turmeric with a pinch black pepper in honey (honeydew honey for kapha) three times a day.
- Apply a warm paste made from long pepper as needed.
- Apply a dry and hot poultice of ajwain seeds as needed.
- Apply a warm paste made from ground fenugreek seeds as needed.
- Apply a paste made from crushed cumin seeds as needed.
- Apply a poultice of tulsi or western basil leaves as needed.
- Apply a hot poultice of dill seeds as needed.
- Massage the affected area with 1 tsp ground ginger or nutmeg mixed with 100ml (3½fl oz) warm sesame oil, or 1 tsp ground fenugreek with 100ml (3½fl oz) mustard oil as needed.
- Take a warm bath containing a dill seed decoction.

Tendinitis

Any dosha can be involved in tendinitis. The best treatment is rest, but you can also use the following remedy. Seek professional medical advice if you are unable to move the joint at all.

FOR ALL DOSHAS

- Apply 1 tbsp grated ginger mixed with 1 tbsp honey to the tender area as needed.

Tired feet

This remedy will ease pain or tiredness in the feet.

FOR ALL DOSHAS

- Take a warm foot bath containing a bay leaf decoction each day.

Wounds

Any wound should be dressed with an antiseptic and, if serious, medical expertise should be sought.

Fresh wounds

Use these remedies to treat wounds immediately after they occur.

FOR ALL DOSHAS

- Sprinkle ground turmeric onto the wound (it is an antiseptic and will stop the bleeding).
- Take ¾ tsp ground turmeric mixed with ½ tsp cane sugar three times a day for up to 3 days (it will dissolve any bruising and reduce swelling and pain).

Old wounds

Use these remedies to treat wounds that are not healing properly as a scab is not forming effectively.

FOR ALL DOSHAS

- Apply a poultice of long pepper with 1 tsp honey (this increases circulation, reduces swelling, and cleans the wound).
- Apply a thin, watered-down paste made from turmeric.
- Apply dry ground turmeric.

Infected wounds

If you think a wound has become infected, seek professional medical advice and use these remedies only if approved by the professional treating you.

FOR ALL DOSHAS

- Apply a paste of ground ajwain in hot water.
- If there are ulcerations, apply fresh mint juice or mint oil up to three times a day.

GLOSSARY **OF TERMS**

agni the digestive fire; it is required to properly digest food, create healthy dhatus (tissues), and produce ojas.

ama undigested food that acts like a toxin. It can be digested (removed) by healthy aqni.

asana a pose that is used as a physical exercise during a yoga session.

ashtanga the classical system by which yoga and meditation are practised. It literally means "eight steps".

Ayurveda the classical Indian medical system; it encompasses healthy living, and preventing and treating disease.

Ayurvedic water water boiled for up to 20 minutes and taken hot. It activates agni (digestive fire) and aids digestion.

brahma muhurta the time at dawn from 4–6am when sattva is dominant. It is particularly good for yoga, meditation, and spiritual practices.

chakra point points on the body that energy can be focused on and channelled through. They are used for practices such as meditation and pranayama.

constitution a person's constitution (or "prakriti" in Sanskrit). It is determined at conception and is the proportions of the three doshas in every individual.

corpse pose the pose used for relaxation during yoga sessions.

dhatus the seven body tissues, these make up the body's physical form.

doshas three energies that make up the body and mind. If unbalanced (minor imbalances called "irritation" and major called "elevation"), they cause ill health.

guna (qualities) literally means "quality" or "characteristic". There are 20 major physical gunas. For the gunas of the mind, *see* three gunas, the.

hatha yoga asanas and pranayama that aid control of prana (life energy), with the aim of controlling the mind.

kapha the dosha that gives substance, cohesion, lubrication, and strength.

malas the body's waste products (stool, urine, sweat).

kapalabhati (lung purification) a yogic breathing exercise.

karma yoga the practice of selflessly serving others.

mantra a phrase or sound that is used for meditation or mantra practice.

nasya the application of oil to the insides of the nostrils either as part of the daily hygiene routine or as a panchakarma treatment.

neti pot a teapot-shaped vessel used to pour salt water into the nostrils to clear the nasal passages and sinuses.

nirguna mantra an abstract mantra relating to the Self.

oil pulling the practice of rinsing the mouth with oil as part of the daily hygiene routine.

ojas the "eighth" tissue, it is one of the substances that anchors prana (life energy) in the body and protects the dhatus from the damaging effects of the doshas.

panchakarma body treatments that cleanse the body of excess doshas.

pitta the dosha that is responsible for all processes of transformation in the body.

prakriti *see* constitution.

prana life energy, required for the body's motor, organ, and sensory functions.

pranayama the practice of energy control through conscious breathing.

rajas (rajasic) one of the three mental gunas. It is the energy of restlessness.

raja yoga exercises that involve mental control and meditation.

rasayana restorative herbal preparations which create healthy dhatus and increase resilience.

saguna mantra a concrete mantra related to a deity.

sattva (sattvic) one of the mental gunas. It is the energy of clarity and harmony.

Self, the this is consciousness (often described as the soul). It is separate from the mind and physical body.

shirodhara a body treatment; oil or buttermilk is poured onto the forehead.

solar plexus the chakra point found behind the stomach.

tamas (tamasic) one of the three mental gunas. It causes inertia and lethargy.

third eye a chakra point found in the centre of the forehead between the eyes.

three gunas, the the three qualities of the mind (sattva, tamas, and rajas).

vata the dosha responsible for all of the body's movement and sensation.

INDEX

A

abdomen 191
   abdominal breathing 40, 124, 125, 160
abhyanga 192, 195
abscesses 210
acid reflux 209
acne 210
adulthood 31
affirmations, positive 173, 185
age 189
agni 13, 26, 188, 214
   daily routines and 32
   digestion and 62
   drinks for 85
   healthy agni 26–27
   hot water and 35
   kapha and 81
   massage oils and 38
   massages when agni is weak 39
   nails and 191
   ojas and 85
   pitta and 77
   the seasons and 31
   strengthening 56–57
   supporting 84–85
   vata and 73
   weak agni 26–27, 49, 209
agni drink 85
ailments
   common 200–201, 204–205
   digestive tract 208–209
   eyes, hair, skin, and teeth 210–11
   respiratory tract 206–207
   trauma and musculoskeletal 212–13
air element 14, 20
alcohol 43
almonds
   almond vegetables 102–103
   kheer 116
aloo methi with mango chutney 106
alternate nostril breathing 126–27
ama 13, 35, 89, 214
   oil massages and 38
   preparing for panchakarma 195
   weak agni and 26
anaemia 204
anxiety 204

appetite loss 208
arishtas 196
aromas, inhaling 35
art 172
artha 8
arthritis 193
asanas 57, 120, 122–23, 214
asavas 196
ashtanga 214
asthma 206
astringent foods 63
autosuggestion, relaxation using 162–63
autumn 31
avocados
   avocado-olive dip 109
   kapha spread 95
   pitta spread 94
   vata spread 94
awareness, of mental state 168–69
Ayurveda practice
   definition of 8, 214
   diagnosis 188–91
Ayurvedic water 85, 214

B

babies, flatulence and bloating
   remedies 209
back, classic oil massage 192
bad breath 204
balance 12, 30
basil 69
basti 194, 195
baths 35, 192
bay leaves 69
beetroot: vata spread 94
bitter foods 63
bloating 209
blocking therapies 193
blood 26
   blood letting 194
   pitta and 201
blood pressure, high 193
the body
   Ayurveda and 12–13
   body awareness 40
   building immunity 26–27

   classic oil massage 192
   daily influence of doshas 31
   kapha body 25
   looking after your body 34–39
   pain remedies 212
   pitta body 23
   treatments 192–93, 195
   vata body 21
bone marrow 26
bones 26, 200
   bone fractures & osteoporosis 212
bowels
   bowel movements 42, 45
   evacuating 35, 194
brahma muhurta 33, 214
breakfast 88, 90–95
   healthier lifestyles and 40, 42, 43
breath, bad 204
breathing
   abdominal 40, 124, 125, 160
   alternate nostril breathing 126–27
   breathing exercises 43
   full yogic breath 125
   lung purification 128–29
   pranayama 120, 122, 124–25
bronchitis 206
burns 212
butter 67

C

caffeine 41
camel 151
cardamom 68
chakras 176, 180, 214
cheese 84
chest 15, 191
childhood 31
children, ailment remedies 206, 207, 208
child's pose 150
chillies 69
cholesterol, high 204
chutney
   ginger-raisin chutney 110
   mango chutney 106
cinnamon 69
cleanliness 34, 174

climate 195
cloves 68
cobra 148–49
coconut: spiced rice vermicelli 90
cold extracts, preparing 202
colds 200, 201, 206
colitis 208
colon 14, 200, 208
compassion 40, 67
complexion 210
concentration, improving 192
conjunctivitis 210
constipation 208
constitution 188, 214
    revealing your 16–19
contentment 174
cooking at home 88–89
coriander 68
corpse pose 160, 214
coughs 206–207
courgettes: baked cumin potatoes with
    courgettes and hummus 98–99
crow 154–55
crumble, fruit 115
cucumber
    pitta spread 94
    raita 101
cumin 69
    baked cumin potatoes with courgettes
    and hummus 98–99
curd 84
curry leaves 69

D

dairy 64, 75, 79, 83, 84
dancing 54
decoctions 196, 202
deep introspection 168, 174
depression 192
desserts 114–17
dhal: simple dhal with grains and
    almond vegetables 102–103
dharma 8, 182
dhatus 13, 26, 188, 214
    strengthening with body
    treatments 192–93
diabetes 201, 204
diagnosis 188–89
diarrhoea 208
diet 189

bronchitis and 206
common colds and 206
constipation and 208
diabetes and 204
diarrhoea and 208
flatulence and bloating and 209
healthy 60–61
indigestion, weak agni and 209
kapha diet 80–81
pacifying kapha 55
pacifying pitta 53
pacifying vata 51
pitta diet 76–77
respiratory tract infection and 207
sattvic diet 64–65
sinus headache and 207
strengthening agni 57
vata diet 72–73
digestion
    improving 84
    remedies for ailments 208–209
    three phases of 62
dinner 88, 108–13
    healthier lifestyles and 40, 41, 42, 43
dip, avocado-olive 109
discipline 175
discs, slipped or worn 193
diseases 48–49
    elevation of doshas and 200
    treating ailments 200–213
doshas 12, 14–15, 214
    daily influence and routine 31, 32–3
    diseases and 48–49
    gunas and 167
    imbalances 188
    pacifying with body treatments
        192–93, 195
    panchakarma and 194
    the seasons and 31
    six tastes and 62–63
    treating common ailments by 200–201
    weak agni and 26
    yoga and the 121
    see also kapha; pitta; vata
drinks 60, 75, 79, 83
    for agni 85
    lassi 117
dry powder massages 38, 193, 195
    kapha and 38, 45, 193
    preparing 39
    strengthening agni 38, 56
drying therapies 193

E

earache 204
earth element 15
the ego 182
elements, doshas and 14–15
emesis 194
enemas 194, 195
ether element 14, 20
exercise
    agni and 56
    healthier lifestyles and 41, 43, 45
    kapha and 54
    pitta and 52
    vata and 50
eyes 191, 201
    eye bath 193
    preserving healthy eyesight 193
    refreshing 35
    remedies for 210
    soothing irritated 45, 193

F

face, classic oil massage 192
fasting 45, 57, 84
    for health 86–87
    vata and 73
fatigue 204
fats 26, 75, 79, 83
feet 192, 213
fennel seeds 68
fenugreek 69
fever 205
fire element 15, 22
fish 142–43
flatulence 209
fluctuations, natural 31
fomentation therapies 193
food
    healing power of 60–61
    healthier lifestyles and 40, 42, 44, 45
    healthy swaps 65
    incompatible foods 61
    for kapha 82–83
    modern food production 67
    nourishing 60
    for pitta 78–79
    purifying 60
    rajasic foods 65

sattvic 64
shopping for 66
tamasic foods 65
for vata 74–75
forehead, oil pouring on the 192, 195
forward bend, sitting 144–45
fritters: vegetable fritters with avocado-
olive dip 109
fruit 64, 75, 79, 83
fruit crumble 115
full yogic breath 125

G

gastritis 209
genital tract 200
ghee 45, 70, 196, 197
inner oiling 195
ginger 68
ginger-raisin chutney 110
goals, setting 9
grains 74, 78, 82
grain porridge 91
simple dhal with grains and almond
vegetables 102–103
gratin, Mediterranean vegetable 96
grounding, vata and 50
gunas 14, 166–67, 214

H

hair loss 210
hardship, comfort in 184
harm, preventing 174
hatha yoga 120, 214
head
classic oil massage 192
heat in the head 205
head colds 200, 201
headaches 192, 205, 207
healing 192
healing power of food 60–61
kapha and 15
health, good 46–57, 66
heart disease 200
heartburn 209
herbs 200
effects on doshas 68
for kapha 83
forms of herbal preparations 196

herbal bolus massage 193, 195
pesto sauce 112
for pitta 79
for vata 75
high blood pressure 193
higher powers, surrendering to 175
hoarseness, sore throat with 207
home remedies 198–213
choosing the right 200
for common ailments 204–13
preparing 202–203
honey 70, 71, 91
hormones, balancing 192
hot flushes 205
hummus 99

I

illness, preventing 188
imbalances, ailments as 200–201
immunity
boosting 192
how the body builds 26–27
inclined plane 146–47
indigestion 209
ingredients, for Ayurvedic remedies 203
inner oiling 195
insect bites & stings 211
insomnia 205
intestines 15, 201
introspection, deep 168, 174
itching 211

J

jaggery 70, 71
joint problems 193, 200
reducing joint stiffness 192
remedies for joint pain 213

K

kama 9
kapalabhati 128–29, 214
kapha 12, 15, 214
active relaxation 161
ailments 201
alternate nostril breathing 126
anxiety remedies 204

balancing 82
camel 151
chanting for 179
chest and 191
childhood and 31
child's pose 150
cobra 148
common cold remedies 206
cough remedies 206–207
crow 154
daily routines and 32, 33
diet 80–81
digestion and 62
elevated 49, 193, 194, 200, 201
elevating 196, 200
eyes and 191
fasting and 87
fish 142
flatulence and bloating remedies 209
foods for 82–83
foods to reduce or avoid 82
gastritis remedies 209
headache remedies 205
healthier lifestyles and 41, 43, 45
herbal bolus massage 193
high cholesterol remedies 204
inclined plane 146
indigestion and weak agni remedies 209
insomnia remedies 205
itching remedies 211
lung purification 128
massage and 37, 39
migraine remedies 205
mind and body 24–25
neck exercises 130
numbness remedies 212
pacifying 54–55, 196
pain remedies 212
panchakarma and 194
plough 140
pranayama 124
pulse and 190
qualities of 24
respiratory tract infection remedies 207
rheumatism remedies 213
shoulderstand 138
single leg lift 136
sinus headache remedies 207
sitting forward bend 144
six tastes and 63
skin and 191, 211
sleep for 33

soothing 195
sore throat remedies 207
spinal twist 156
spring and 31
sun salutation 132
teeth remedies 211
tongue and 191
tree 152
triangle 158
winter and 31
yoga and 121, 123
kapha spread 95
karma yoga 182–83, 214
Kerala panchakarma 194, 195
kheer 116
khichdi with raita 100–101

L

lassi 117
leech therapy 194
leg lifts, single 136–37
legumes 64
lentils: khichdi with raita 100–101
life, phases of 31
lifestyle 189
    healthy 30–31, 40–45
    pacifying kapha 54
    pacifying pitta 52
    pacifying vata 50
    strengthening agni 56
limb pain 213
liver, pitta and 201
long pepper 68, 203
lozenges, preparing 203
lumbago 193, 212
lunch 60, 88, 96–107
    healthier lifestyles and 40, 42
lung purification 128–29

M

malas 12, 26, 189, 214
mango chutney 106
mantras 180–81, 214
    power of 178–79
massage 40
    agni and 56
    dry powder massage 38, 39, 45, 56,
       193, 195

herbal bolus massage 193, 195
    kapha and 54
    oil massage 35, 45, 50, 192, 195
    pitta and 52
    self-massage 36–37, 42, 43, 44
    vata and 50
massage oils, choosing 38–39
meals 43
    guidelines 85
    mealtimes 32, 40, 42, 44, 60, 88
meat 67
medicines, Ayurvedic 196–97
meditation 176–79
    healthier lifestyles and 40, 42, 43, 44
    pacifying kapha 55
    pacifying pitta 53
    pacifying vata 51
Mediterranean vegetable gratin 96
menstrual pain 193
mental health see mind
metabolism 45, 54, 201
migraines 205
milk 45, 67
    kheer 116
the mind
    and autosuggestion 163
    Ayurveda and the 166–67
    benefits of mantras 178, 179
    kapha mind 24
    karma yoga 182–83
    keeping healthy 166
    mental relaxation 162
    monitoring the mind 168–69
    pitta mind 22
    the Self and 170–71
    state of mind 168–69, 188
    ultimate mental health 184–5
    vata mind 20
mint 68
moderation 30
modest living 175
moksha 8, 9, 184
motivation 168
mouth ulcers 207
movement 15
mucous 191
mung dhal 99
muscles 26
musculoskeletal ailments, remedies
    for 212–13
music 172
mustard seeds 69

N

nails 191
nasal passages
    clearing 35, 40
    nasya 34, 42, 45, 194, 214
nausea 209
neck exercises 42, 130–31, 143
negative thoughts 166
nervous system
    calming 192
    nerve pain 193
    nerve tissue 26
neti pots 35, 214
nirguna mantras 180, 214
noodles, sesame 105
nosebleeds 205
nostrils, oiling 194
nourishment 66
    nourishing foods 60
    nourishing therapies 193
numbness 212
nutmeg 69
nuts 64, 75, 79, 83
    pesto sauce 112
    spiced rice vermicelli 90

O

oil massages 35, 45, 50, 192, 195
oil pulling 34, 42, 214
oiling therapies 193
    inner oiling 195
    local oil treatment 193
    oil pouring on the forehead
       192, 195
    oiling nostrils 194
oils, herbal 196
ojas 188, 214
    agni and 26, 85
    dhatus 13, 177
    immunity and 26, 27, 188
old age 31
olives: avocado-olive dip 109
OM sound 180
oregano 69
organic food 66
osteoarthritis 212
osteoporosis 212
overeating 89

P

pain
    alleviating 192
    joints & limb pain 213
    remedies for 212
pancakes, wholegrain 92
panchakarma 45, 194–95, 214
parsley 69
pasta: wholegrain pasta with pesto
        sauce 112
pastes, preparing 202
peas: spiced rice vermicelli 90
pesto sauce 112
pills, preparing 203
pippali 68, 203
pitta 12, 15, 214
    active relaxation 161
    adulthood and 31
    ailments and 201
    alternate nostril breathing 126
    anxiety remedies 204
    balancing 78
    camel 151
    chanting for 179
    child's pose 150
    cobra 148
    common cold remedies 206
    constipation remedies 208
    cough remedies 207
    crow 154
    daily routines and 32, 33
    diet 76–77
    digestion and 62
    elevated 48, 49, 194, 195, 200, 201
    elevating 196, 200
    eyes and 191, 210
    fasting and 87
    fish 142
    foods for 78–79
    foods to reduce or avoid 78
    gastritis remedies 209
    healthier lifestyles and 41, 43, 45
    herbal bolus massage 193
    hot flushes remedies 205
    inclined plane 146
    indigestion and weak agni
        remedies 209
    insomnia remedies 205
    lung purification 128
    massage oils 38

    massages for 38
    mind and body 22–23
    neck exercises 130
    pacifying 52–53, 196
    pain remedies 212
    panchakarma and 194
    plough 140
    pranayama 124
    pulse and 190
    qualities of 22
    respiratory tract infection
        remedies 207
    rheumatism remedies 213
    shoulderstand 138
    single leg lift 136
    sitting forward bend 144
    six tastes and 63
    skin and 191
    sleep for 33
    soothing 195
    spinal twist 156
    summer and 31
    sun salutation 132
    tiredness remedies 204
    tongue and 191
    tree 152
    triangle 158
    yoga and 121, 123
pitta spread 94
plants, healing power of 201
plasma 26
plough 140–41
porridge, grain 91
positive thinking 40, 42, 164–75
potatoes
    aloo methi 106
    baked cumin potatoes with courgettes
        and hummus 98–99
potency 196
poultices, preparing 203
prana 214
    and balance 12
    ojas and 13, 26, 27
pranayama 124–25, 214
    healthier lifestyles and 42
    tips 122
    and yoga 120
problems, recognizing 48–49
processed food 60
prunes: tridosha spread 95
psyllium husk 203
pulao, rice 110

pulse 190
pulses 75, 79, 83
pungent foods 63
purgation 194, 195
purification
    purifying foods 60, 103
    purifying therapies 194

Q

qualities 196

R

raisins
    ginger-raisin chutney 110
    grain porridge 91
raita 101
raja yoga 120, 163, 164–85, 214
rajas 65, 166, 167, 168, 214
    rajasic foods 65
rakta moksha 194
rasayana 197, 214
rashes 211
raw foods 96
reducing therapies 193
regional food 60
relaxation 120, 121
    active relaxation 41, 160–61
    finishing 163
    mental 162
    physical 162
    shirodhara and 192
    spiritual 163
    tips 123
    using autosuggestion 162–63
remedies, home 45, 198–213
    choosing the right 200
    for common ailments 204–13
    preparing 202–203
reproductive tissue 26
respiratory tract
    kapha and 201
    remedies for ailments 206–207
restorative medicines 197
rheumatism 213
rheumatoid arthritis 213
rice
    kheer 116
    khichdi with raita 100–101

rice pulao with ginger-raisin chutney 110
ricotta cheese: pesto sauce 112
rocket: kapha spread 95
rosemary 69
routines 30
    daily 32–33, 43
    morning 34–35, 40, 42, 44
runny nose 207

S

saffron 68
saguna mantras 181, 214
salads 96
    crisp salad with sunflower-lemon dressing 97
salt 62, 75, 79, 83
sattva 214
    gaining with our actions 174
    healthier lifestyles and 42
    and the mind 166
    positive thinking 172
    sattvic diet 64–65, 66
sciatica 212
seasons
    food and 60
    strength of agni and doshas during 31
seeds 64, 75, 79, 83
    spiced rice vermicelli 90
the Self 214
    awareness of 184
    the mind and 170–71
    and modest living 175
    separating from the mind 170–71
self-assessment questionnaire 16–19
self-improvement 175
sensation
    sensory pleasure 9, 172
    vata and 15
sesame noodles 105
sexuality, moderation in 175
sharkara 70, 71
shirodhara 192, 214
shoulderstand 138–39
showers 35, 42
single leg lift 136–37
sinus headaches 207
sitting forward bend 144–45

skin 26, 191
    dry, cracked 211
    irritation or rashes 211
    pitta and 201
    remedies for 210
sleep 32
    improving 33, 41, 43, 192
    insomnia 205
SO'HAM mantra 180
solar plexus 125, 214
soothing 192
sore throats 207
soups
    creamy squash soup 107
    mixed vegetable soup 111
sour foods 62
spices 44, 200
    effects on doshas 69
    for kapha 83
    for pitta 79
    sattvic foods 64
    spiced rice vermicelli 90
    strengthening agni 57
    for vata 75
spinal twist 156–57
spiritual relaxation 163
sprains 213
spreads, breakfast 94–95
spring 31
squash: creamy squash soup 107
stealing 175
steam baths 192
stir-fried vegetables with sesame noodles 104–105
stomach
    gastritis with stomach pain 209
    kapha and 15, 201
    pitta and 15, 201
stools 26
strength, physical 189
    strength-building exercises 50
sugar 43, 70, 71, 197
summer 31
sun salutation 132–35
sunflower seeds: grain porridge 91
sweat 26
sweet foods 62
sweeteners 64, 75, 79, 83
swelling, joints & limbs 213
swimming 52

T

tamas 65, 166, 167, 168, 214
taste
    Ayurvedic medicines 196
    post-digestive 197
    six tastes 62–63
technology 41, 172
teeth 34, 211
tendinitis 213
third eye 214
thoughts, positive 164–75
the three gunas 214
throat problems 207
tiredness 204
tissues 13
    restoring tissue health 197
    see also dhatus
tolerance 45
tongue 191
    cleaning 34, 40
transformation
    agni and 26
    pitta and 15
trauma
    remedies for 212–13
    vata and 200
travel 195
tree 152–53
triangle 158–59
tridosha spread 95
truthfulness 174
tulsi 203
turmeric 68

U

urinary tract 200, 205
urine 26

V

values, refining 174–75
vamana 194
vata 12, 14, 214
    active relaxation 161
    ailments 200
    alternate nostril breathing 126

anxiety remedies 204
autumn and 31
balancing 64
camel 151
chanting for 179
child's pose 150
cobra 148
common cold remedies 206
constipation remedies 208
cough remedies 206–207
crow 154
daily routines and 32, 33
diet 72–73
digestion and 62
elevated 48, 49, 194, 195, 200
elevating 196, 200
eyes and 191, 210
fasting and 87
fish 142
flatulence and bloating
    remedies 209
foods for 74–75
foods to reduce or avoid 74
gastritis remedies 209
headache remedies 205
healthier lifestyles and 41, 43, 45
herbal bolus massage 193
high cholesterol remedies 204
hot flushes remedies 205
inclined plane 146
indigestion and weak agni
    remedies 209
insomnia remedies 205
itching remedies 211
lung purification 128
massage and 38, 50
migraine remedies 205
mind and body 20–21
neck exercises 130
numbness remedies 212
oil massages and 192
old age and 31
pacifying 50–51, 193, 196
pain remedies 212
plough 140
pranayama 124
pulse and 190
qualities of 20
respiratory tract infection
    remedies 207
rheumatism remedies 213

shoulderstand 138
single leg lift 136
sinus headache remedies 207
sitting forward bend 144
six tastes and 63
skin and 191, 211
sleep for 33
soothing 195
sore throat remedies 207
spinal twist 156
sun salutation 132
teeth remedies 211
tiredness remedies 204
tongue and 191
tree 152
triangle 158
winter and 31
yoga and 121, 123
vata spread 94
vegetables 64, 75, 79, 83
    almond vegetables 102–103
    khichdi with raita 100–101
    Mediterranean vegetable gratin 96
    mixed vegetable soup 111
    rice pulao 110
    stir-fried vegetables with sesame
    noodles 104–105
    vegetable fritters with avocado-olive
    dip 109
vegetarianism 42, 44, 66–67
vermicelli, spiced rice 90
virechana 194, 195
voice loss 207
vomiting, therapeutic 194

W

walks 172
warm up 122
water
    Ayurvedic water 214
    cold water 84
    hot water 35, 40, 42, 43, 60
water element 15, 22
wealth, material 8
weight loss 205
weightlifting 50
whole grains 64
wines, herbal 196
winter 31

work 43
wounds 213

Y

yoga 118–63
    Ayurveda and 8–9
    constipation remedies 208
    diabetes remedies 204
    hatha yoga 214
    healthier lifestyles and 40, 42, 44
    indigestion and weak agni
        remedies 209
    karma yoga 182–83, 214
    pacifying kapha 55
    pacifying pitta 53
    pacifying vata 51
    raja yoga 163, 214
    strengthening agni 57
    your yoga session 122–23
yogurt 84
    lassi 117
    raita 101

INTERNATIONAL SIVANANDA YOGA VEDANTA CENTRES AND ASHRAMS

Centres offer classes and workshops in asanas, pranayama, meditation, vegetarian cooking and Ayurveda, yoga psychology and philosophy, yoga vacation programmes, and teachers' training courses.

Founded by:
SWAMI VISHNUDEVANANDA

www.sivananda.org

Headquarters

CANADA
Sivananda Ashram Yoga Camp
673, 8th Avenue Val Morin
Quebec J0T 2R0,
Canada

www.sivananda.org/camp

Ashrams

AUSTRIA
Sivananda Yoga Retreat House
Bichlach 40
A- 6370 Reith bei Kitzbühel
Tyrol, Austria

www.sivananda.at

BAHAMAS
Sivananda Ashram Yoga Retreat
P.O. Box N7550 Paradise Island
Nassau,
Bahamas

www.sivanandabahamas.org

FRANCE
Château du Yoga Sivananda
26 Impasse du Bignon
45170 Neuville aux bois,
France

www.sivanandaorleans.org

INDIA
Sivananda Yoga Vedanta
Meenakshi Ashram
Near Pavanna Vilakku Junction,
New Natham Road
Saramthangi Village
Madurai Dist. 625 503
Tamil Nadu, South India

www.sivananda.org/madurai

Sivananda Kutir
(Near Siror Bridge)
P.O. Netala, Uttar Kashi Dt.
Uttarakhand, Himalayas, 249 193,
North India

www.sivananda.org/netala

Sivananda Yoga Vedanta
Dhanwantari Ashram
P.O. Neyyar Dam
Thiruvananthapuram Dt.
Kerala, 695 572, India

www.sivananda.org/neyyardam

International Sivananda Yoga Vedanta
Tapaswini Ashram
Guthavaripalem, Kadivedu P.O.
Chilakur Mandalam, Gudur, India

www.sivananda.org.in/gudur

UNITED STATES
Sivananda Ashram Yoga Ranch
P.O. Box 195, 500 Budd Road
Woodbourne, NY 12788, USA

www.sivanandayogaranch.org

Sivananda Ashram Yoga Farm
14651 Ballantree Lane
Grass Valley, CA 95949, USA

www.sivanandayogafarm.org

VIETNAM
Sivananda Yoga Vietnam Resort and Training Centre
K'Lan Eco Resort, Tuyen Lam Lake;
Dalat, Vietnam

www.sivanandayogavietnam.org

Centres

ARGENTINA
Centro Internaciónal de Yoga Sivananda
Sánchez de Bustamante 2372 -
(C.P. 1425)
Capital Federal - Buenos Aires -Argentina

www.sivananda.org/buenosaires

Centro de Yoga Sivananda
Rioja 425, 8300 Neuquén, Argentina

www.facebook.com/SivanandaNeuquen/

AUSTRIA
Sivananda Yoga Vedanta Zentrum
Prinz Eugen Strasse 18
A -1040 Vienna, Austria

www.sivananda.org/vienna

BRAZIL
Centro Sivananda de Yoga Vedanta
Rua Santo Antônio 374, Bairro Floresta
Porto Alegre 90220-010, Brazil

www.sivananda.org/portoalegre

Centro International Sivananda de Yoga e Vedanta
Rua Girassol 1088, Vila Madalena
Sao Paulo 05433-002, Brazil

www.sivananda.org/saopaulo

CANADA
Sivananda Yoga Vedanta Centre
5178 St Lawrence Blvd, Montreal,
Quebec H2T 1R8, Canada
www.sivananda.org/montreal

Sivananda Yoga Vedanta Centre
77 Harbord Street
Toronto, Ontario M5S 1G4, Canada
www.sivananda.org/toronto

CHINA
Sivananda Yoga Vedanta Center
Zhonghuayuan Xiuyuan 30-3-202,
5 Tongzilin East Road,
Wuhou District, Chengdu, Sichuan
610041 China
www.sivanandayogachina.org

FRANCE
Centre Sivananda de Yoga Vedanta
140 rue du Faubourg Saint-Martin
F-75010 Paris
France
www.sivananda.org/paris

GERMANY
Sivananda Yoga Vedanta Zentrum
Steinheilstrasse 1
D-80333 Munich, Germany
www.sivananda.org/munich

Sivananda Yoga Vedanta Zentrum
Schmiljanstrasse 24
D-12161 Berlin, Germany
www.sivananda.org/berlin

INDIA
Sivananda Yoga Vedanta Nataraja Centre
A-41 Kailash Colony
New Delhi 110 048, India
www.sivananda.org/delhi

Sivananda Yoga Vedanta Dwarka Centre
(near DAV school, next to Kamakshi Apts)
PSP Pocket, Sector – 6

Swami Sivananda Marg,
Dwarka, New Delhi 110 075,

India
www.sivananda.org/dwarka

Sivananda Yoga Vedanta Centre
TC37/1927 (5), Airport Road, West Fort P.O.
Thiruvananthapuram
Kerala 695 023, India
www.sivananda.org/trivandrum

Sivananda Yoga Vedanta Centre
3/655 (Plot No. 131) Kaveri Nagar
Kuppam Road, Kottivakkam
Chennai, Tamil Nadu 600 041, India
www.sivananda.org/chennai

Sivananda Yoga Vedanta Centre
444, K.K. Nagar, East 9th Street
Madurai, Tamil Nadu 625 020, India
www.sivananda.org/maduraicentre

ISRAEL
Sivananda Yoga Vedanta Centre
6 Lateris St, Tel Aviv 64166, Israel
www.sivananda.co.il

ITALY
Centro Yoga Vedanta Sivananda Roma
Via Oreste Tommasini, 7
00162 Rome, Italy
www.sivananda-yoga-roma.it

Centro Yoga Vedanta Sivananda
Milano, Milan, Italy
Phone: +39.334.760.5376
e-mail: Milan@sivananda.org

JAPAN
Sivananda Yoga Vedanta Centre
4-15-3 Koenji-kita, Suginami-ku
Tokyo 1660002, Japan
www.sivananda.jp

LITHUANIA
**Šivananda Yogos Vedantos Centras
Vilniuje**
M.K. Čiurlionio g. 66, 03100 Vilnius
Lithuania
www.sivananda.org/vilnius

SPAIN
Centro de Yoga Sivananda Vedanta
Calle Eraso 4, 28028 Madrid
www.sivananda.org/madrid

SWITZERLAND
Centre Sivananda de Yoga Vedanta
1 Rue des Minoteries
1205 Geneva, Switzerland
www.sivananda.org/geneva

UNITED KINGDOM
Sivananda Yoga Vedanta Centre
45–51 Felsham Road
London SW15 1AZ, UK
www.sivananda.co.uk

UNITED STATES
Sivananda Yoga Vedanta Center
1246 West Bryn Mawr
Chicago, IL 60660, USA
www.sivanandachicago.org

Sivananda Yoga Vedanta Center
243 West 24th Street
New York, NY 10011, USA
www.sivanandanyc.org

Sivananda Yoga Vedanta Center
1185 Vicente Street
San Francisco, CA 94116, USA
www.sivanandasf.org

Sivananda Yoga Vedanta Center
13325 Beach Avenue
Marina del Rey, CA 90292, USA
www.sivanandala.org

URUGUAY
Asociación de Yoga Sivananda
Acevedo Díaz 1523
11200 Montevideo, Uruguay
www.sivananda.org/montevideo

VIETNAM
Sivananda Yoga Vedanta Centre
25 Tran Quy Khoach Street, District 1
Ho Chi Minh City, Vietnam
www.sivanandayogavietnam.org

ABOUT THE AUTHORS

Yoga Acharyas, members of the board of directors of the International Sivananda Yoga Vedanta Centres, and senior teachers of the Sivananda Yoga Teachers' Training Courses:

SWAMI DURGANANDA

Swami Durgananda established the Sivananda Yoga Vedanta Centres in Europe on the request of her teacher Swami Vishnudevananda. Swami Durgananda has taught several generations of yoga students, as well as teachers, about how to apply the principles of Ayurveda and yoga in order to practise a healthy and spiritual way of life. Her vision and advice is the guiding thread of this book. swd@sivananda.net

SWAMI SIVADASANANDA

Swami Sivadasananda compiled the chapter on asana, pranayama, and relaxation based on the teaching system and the practical inspiration of his teacher Swami Vishnudevananda. He teaches courses and workshops around the world with profound knowledge and a dynamic and precise teaching style. sws@sivananda.net

SWAMI KAILASANANDA

A senior disciple of Swami Vishnudevananda, Swami Kailasananda shares her many years of dedicated practice and teaching experience in the meditation section of this book. swk@sivananda.net

The board members would like to thank the other contributing members of the International Sivananda Yoga Vedanta Centres:

CORDULA INTERTHAL

We would like to thank Cordula Interthal (Chandrika) for her dedication in writing the chapters on the body, Ayurvedic lifestyle, maintaining health, food, visiting an Ayurvedic practitioner, and home remedies. Cordula lives in Munich, Germany, where she combines her talents as medical doctor, Ayurvedic practitioner, and yoga teacher. www.devi-ayurveda.de

SWAMI BHAGAVATANANDA

We would like to thank Swami Bhagavatananda, a senior teacher of the Sivananda Yoga Vedanta Centres, for the skillful compilation of the recipe section. swb@sivananda.net

ACKNOWLEDGMENTS

AUTHORS' ACKNOWLEDGMENTS

We would like to thank Ayurveda-Acharya Shanti Kumar Kamlesh from Lucknow, India, for sharing his practical and enthusiastic knowledge of Ayurvedic diet and lifestyle during countless visits in the Sivananda Centres during the past 20 years.

Cordula would like to thank the Seva Academy in Munich, and especially her Ayurveda teacher Dr Neelesh Taware, for generously sharing their knowledge and expertise.

PUBLISHER'S ACKNOWLEDGMENTS

The publisher would like to thank Soma Chowdhury, Janashree Singha, Madhurika Bhardwaj, and Nonita Saha for their help editing the recipes, Corinne Masciocchi for proofreading, and Vanessa Bird for creating the index.

PICTURE CREDITS

The publisher would like to thank the following for their kind permission to reproduce their photographs:

(Key: a-above; b-below/bottom; c-centre; f-far; l-left; r-right; t-top)

123RF.com: Liudmila Horvath 1c, 2-3, 4-5, 6t, 7r, 8-9, 10-11, 12-13, 14t, 16t, 19t, 20-21t, 21br, 23br, 25br, 27t, 27r, 28-29, 31r, 34bl, 36tr, 39r, 40-41c, 42-43c, 44-45c, 48-49, 50-51, 52-53, 54-55, 56-57, 58-59, 60-61, 64t, 65br, 66b, 67br, 68-69, 72bl, 72-73c, 73t, 75, 76bl, 76-77c, 77t, 79, 80bl, 80-81c, 81t, 83, 84bc, 84-85t, 84-85c, 85br, 86bc, 87tc, 88-89, 90-91, 92-93, 94-95, 96tl, 96bl, 98-99, 100-101, 102-103, 104tl, 104bl, 105tr, 106-107, 108bl, 109, 110-111, 112, 113tr, 114bl, 115, 116-117, 118-119, 122-123t, 122-123c, 123br, 124tr, 125tr, 128tr, 129tr, 130tr, 131tc, 132tr, 134-135t, 136tr, 138tr, 140tr, 141t, 142tr, 144tr, 145cr, 146tr, 148tr, 149tc, 150tr, 151tr, 152tr, 153br, 154tr, 156tr, 158tr, 162-163t, 162-163c, 162-163b, 164-165, 168-169t, 169br, 176tr, 176b, 176-177t, 177br, 178tr, 178-179b, 179, 182b, 183tr, 185tr, 186-187, 189br, 192t, 192bl, 193br, 194t, 194bl, 195br, 198-199, 202-203, 204tr, 205br, 206tr, 207br, 208tr, 209br, 210tr, 211br, 212tr, 217t, 217r, 219t, 219r, 221r, 222-223t, 223br, 224tr, 224cr, Natbasil 22-23t, 191tr, Snezh 24-25t, 30-31, 46-47, 197br, 200-201, 202b, 203t

All other images © Dorling Kindersley

For further information see: www.dkimages.com